'Ed Novak is one of the most exciting contributors to the field of transactional analysis in the world today. This latest offering – an integration of embodied therapy with psychoanalysis and transactional analysis is a wonderful, courageous, provocative invitation to extend the methodology of talking therapy into work that directly engages with embodied trauma. Novak describes the life-limiting embodied effects of trauma and introduces five categories of therapeutic touch, designed to help clients reclaim their 'stolen body'. The book is written with enormous care and thought, including accounting for every type of professional or personal resistance to the idea of touch in therapy, and the style of writing mirrors the evident care, thought and generosity for clients that shine through in the many rich case studies.'

Professor Charlotte Sills, *Integrative Psychotherapist; Teaching and Supervising Transactional Analyst*

'Ever since the mid-1950's, when psychoanalysts began to discuss the "widening scope of psychoanalysis," the field has been beset by the challenges of doing deep and effective treatment with those whose core issues come out of unrepresented and unformulated experience, generally traumatic, with its dissociated or split-off content, often unavailable to memory, but inscribed into the body. Novak offers here a fresh and fearless contribution to the field with his clear, disciplined, and clinically focused approach to psychoanalytic work with the body-mind in which touch can be an essential component.'

David V. Orbison, *Ph.D., Clinical Psychoanalyst in Pittsburgh; Founding Member, KOWA*

'Massage therapists interact with the powerful, undeniable subject of transference and countertransference connections with our clients. Given trauma informed care is the new standard, we are instinctively aware of these connections, but have little information available on how to address them when they surface during a massage. In his book Novak shares his wisdom gathered over decades to expand our curiosity and give vital insight to a subject often viewed in a repressive, dismissive way in massage therapy education. Novak's work opens a new horizon to engage the link between trauma and touch in massage therapy.'

Dorothy Adams, *LMT, Akron, Ohio*

'I became aware of the healing power of touch for severely traumatized and dying patients during the AIDS crisis in New York. I learned that a hand resting on a shoulder or held for a few moments in parting or wrapping a young man in a blanket who is shivering with illness comforts but also evokes memories and feelings that are essential to good therapeutic work. Novak offers us, finally, a safe, systematic and developmentally grounded theory that integrates physical touch with psychoanalytic therapy. Rich with clinical process, the book is a must read for anyone in the mental health fields and everyone interested in how bodies that have been "stolen" can actually be recovered.'

Sandra Kiersky, *Ph.D., Faculty and supervisor, Institute for the Psychoanalytic Study of Subjectivity, New York*

Physical Touch in Psychoanalytic Psychotherapy

This groundbreaking book presents a new model for incorporating the human body, and specifically physical touch, into psychoanalysis and psychotherapy, particularly for patients who have experienced trauma.

Novak's model of informed and disciplined touch articulates five categories of touch and three phases of therapeutic body work, all of which can help move the patient and therapist directly into bodily experiences that enable trauma memories to be processed, and then analyzed and transformed. This transformation leads to patients experiencing their bodies in fundamentally new ways, both relationally and intrapsychically. The book also grapples with the risks and ethics of working directly with patients' bodies, outlining theoretical and clinical elements that help create a safe and sacred therapeutic structure. Novak's model offers a continuum of touch from everyday physical interactions, such as handshakes or hugs, to more complex and complete ways of working with the body that are safe and meaningful and that create an integrated experience of the patient's mind and body.

Physical Touch in Psychoanalytic Psychotherapy is of interest to therapists at all levels of experience in the fields of counseling, social work, psychotherapy, and psychoanalysis. Practitioners in other helping professions such as healthcare, massage therapy, and physical therapy, as well as providers of wholistic medicine, will also be able to make use of the comprehensive clinical model and case studies detailed in the book.

Edward T. Novak is a psychoanalyst in private practice in Akron, Ohio, who trained at the National Institute for the Psychotherapies in their National Training Program in New York. He has presented at international conferences and published numerous articles, including a number on touch in psychotherapy and psychoanalysis. He is the book review editor for the *Transactional Analysis Journal* and a member of the editorial review board.

Physical Touch in Psychoanalytic Psychotherapy

Transforming Trauma through Embodied Practice

Edward T. Novak

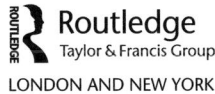

Routledge
Taylor & Francis Group

LONDON AND NEW YORK

Cover image: Getty Images

First published 2023
by Routledge
4 Park Square, Milton Park, Abingdon, Oxon OX14 4RN

and by Routledge
605 Third Avenue, New York, NY 10158

Routledge is an imprint of the Taylor & Francis Group, an informa business

British Library Cataloguing-in-Publication Data
A catalogue record for this book is available from the British Library

Library of Congress Cataloging-in-Publication Data
Names: Novak, Edward T., author.
Title: Physical touch in psychoanalytic psychotherapy : transforming trauma through embodied practice / Edward T. Novak.
Description: Abingdon, Oxon ; New York, NY : Routledge, 2022. | Includes bibliographical references and index. |
Identifiers: LCCN 2022005574 | ISBN 9781032105291 (hardback) |
ISBN 9781032105284 (paperback) | ISBN 9781003215745 (ebook)
Subjects: LCSH: Touch--Therapeutic use. | Touch--Psychological aspects. |
Psychotherapy. | Psychoanalysis.
Classification: LCC RC489.T69 N68 2022 | DDC 616.89/14--dc23/eng/
20220505
LC record available at https://lccn.loc.gov/2022005574

ISBN: 978-1-032-10529-1 (hbk)
ISBN: 978-1-032-10528-4 (pbk)
ISBN: 978-1-003-21574-5 (ebk)

DOI: 10.4324/9781003215745

Typeset in Times New Roman
by Taylor & Francis Books

To Laura and Thomas

Contents

Acknowledgments

"You need to write about this." A persistent and repetitive response from my psychoanalyst whenever I discussed my personal embodied work or consulted my embodied work with one of my patients with her. For over ten years I heard this refrain from Sandra Kiersky as we collaboratively discussed my work and my belief of the essential importance of physical contact for individuals with embodied trauma. Her belief and encouragement that my ideas and work with trauma needed to be published was instrumental in managing my anxieties around publishing this model of embodied therapy. Her teachings and writings on many topics and theories including mother–infant research, attachment theory, and empathic attunement within the theory of self psychology enhanced the theoretical basis of my model. Sandra's own curiosity and independent ideas around therapeutic touch contributed greatly to the clarification of many concepts of this model. Most importantly, Sandra was never judgmental or concerned that my work was too radical. Without her encouragement and support this book would not have been written and for this I am beyond grateful.

For many years supportive colleagues have read and discussed this model in ways that also clarified my thinking and ideas. Within my transactional analysis community, I would like to especially thank Cristina Caizzi, Diana Deaconu, Alexandra Gheorghe, Laurie Hawkes, Mick Landaiche, Sharon Davis Massey, Karen Minikin, Sylvie Monin, Trudi Newton, Steff Oates, Helen Rowland, Charlotte Sills, and Jo Stuthridge.

Within my psychoanalytic community I want to thank Kenneth Frank for his encouragement and support of the first drafts of my model during my psychoanalytic training in the National Institute for the Psychotherapies Training Institute's National Training Program. Other psychoanalysts that have been encouraging of my ideas around embodied therapy have included Maurice Apprey, Howard Bacal, Mario Fischetti, and David Orbison. I also want to thank Doris Brothers and Jon Sletvold for inviting me to present with them and Karen Starr in a seminar that addressed touch in therapy at the 2019 International Association for Relational Psychoanalysis and Psychotherapy (IARPP) conference in New York City. Other supportive colleagues and friends include:

Colleen Denholm, Shane Gamble, Barb Havens, Troy Havens, George Herrity, Chris Meyer, Douglas Roach, Thomas Rock, and Jeff Stetz. My apologies and thanks to those colleagues and friends I may have unintentionally omitted from this group.

For over 20 years I was fortunate to have been in individual consultations with William Cornell along with a study group that also included Claudette Kulkarni, Sally Donnelly, Akiko Motomura, Harry Ritter, and others over that 20-year span. Our group studies and consultations included exploring somatic issues of our patients and the use of touch with specific patients.

A special thank you to Lauren Wylie LMT who was my massage therapist for five years. Our work which is detailed in Chapter 3 was instrumental in my recovery of my own stolen body and the development of this embodied therapy model.

Thank you to Robin Fryer who has been editor, writing mentor, colleague, and friend for almost all of my published works. Robin has advanced my professional writing skills and helped me create my own personal writing style. My appreciation of her enthusiastic willingness to join me in the preparation of the draft of this manuscript and editing each chapter for submission is impossible to language with words.

Thank you to the concealed patients in this book who were courageous enough to engage in embodied work and who enthusiastically granted me permission to discuss and write about their work with me in hopes that others may benefit from it. You have my deep gratitude.

I am privileged to have been offered this opportunity to publish through Routledge and was fortunate to work with several talented professionals throughout the publishing process. My sincere thanks and appreciation to Alexis O'Brien, Katie Randall, Eleonora Kouneni, and Susannah Frearson.

I dedicate this book to my wife Laura and my son Thomas. Laura was saintly in tolerating my chronic obsession with discussing this book while offering meaningful feedback and encouragement throughout the process. Thomas was also supportive and indulgent of my work, including allowing me to practice my massage techniques on him during my brief massage training. Thank you, love, and a meaningful hug to both of you.

Introduction

"I understand. Now what do we do to change this?" Many of my patients asked this question when they realized they could no longer ignore their body in their attempts to work through their abuse and trauma. Despite months, if not years, of hard work on their trauma through talk therapy, the treatment had limited impact on the anxieties and fears around physical contact that continued to limit their life. Although our work had resulted in some changes, the remaining level of embodied trauma was still insufferable. It typically took months, usually years, for the patient to reach the point of asking this question, and it signaled their readiness to directly focus on their traumatized body. The patient's curiosity and courage evoked feelings of both promise and trepidation in me because I then had to decide how to answer. To go further into addressing and transforming their embodied trauma would require working with direct physical contact either with me or someone else.

The problem was that my way of working involved psychoanalysis and psychotherapy that paid primary attention to the mind and the emotions rather than the body, even when working with embodied trauma. Although the body and somatic issues certainly could be addressed, that was almost always done without touch. The possibility of physical touch between patient and therapist received little encouragement or support, if not outright scorn, within the profession. I faced a serious professional dilemma: to include or not include physical contact in the work.

This question paralleled my personal therapeutic journey of over 30 years, which had included therapy that addressed not only the mental and emotional issues of my embodied traumas but my physical body as well. As will be detailed in Chapter 3, this integrated work created transformations for me at both mental and physical levels that have been life changing. Limiting the work to either talk therapy or bodywork alone could never have achieved that.

Back to my patients' question: "What do we do to change this?" Whenever a patient achieved this level of insight and understanding, I experienced an internal conflict between playing it "safe" and avoiding touch or offering the possibility of some form of embodied therapy. I knew they needed someone

DOI: 10.4324/9781003215745-1

with whom to work through their embodied trauma not only with talk but also with touch, someone with whom they could not only do the important work of listening and witnessing their trauma, but also to physically connect to their embodied trauma memories, including their embodied trauma flashbacks. This was what I had created for myself in my own treatment, and I had to consider whether I could offer that experience to my patients as well.

The dilemma was intense, but I knew the incredible transformations that could take place within embodied therapy. Despite my trepidation, I would often offer the patient the choice of including physical touch in their treatment. Not all patients accepted the offer, but those who did greatly benefitted from various forms of body psychotherapy. In my early years of working that way, I was able to provide patients with some techniques that created embodied changes and provided symptom relief that they found deeply important.

It would be over two decades before I had enough training, personal therapy, and embodied therapy to offer my patients more than some embodied change and symptom relief. In my third decade as a psychoanalyst, I began offering patients not only my mind but my physical touch in their analysis when and as appropriate. We engaged in a form of body analysis that was similar to the forms of embodied therapy I had found outside my own personal analysis. The combination of psychoanalysis and body analysis created unimagined transformations for patients in both mind and body. My 30 years of exploring the body and physical touch in fostering psychological well-being both as a clinician and a patient led to my being able to offer a continuum of embodied therapy from symptom relief to body analysis based on the patient's trauma issues as well as their curiosity, consent, readiness, and the therapeutic fit between us (Bacal, 2011).

For patients who choose not to include direct physical touch in their work with me, I help them explore their body issues using bodywork they secure outside of our work. For instance, some patients work with massage therapists, yoga practitioners, and so on, and then bring their experiences back to the analysis for processing, much as I had done in my own therapy.

Some patients are not convinced of the importance of attending to their body in treatment. In fact, most of them have spent years dealing with and defending against feelings of having been terrorized at a body level. For them, it is too difficult to commit to bodywork in any capacity. In such cases, we work to find levels of repair in nontouch therapy, paying attention to their body through discussions.

In 2017, I presented my model of touch in therapy along with a case example at a transactional analysis conference in Berlin, Germany. The presentation was a 3-hour paper given in a small classroom designed for 35 students. On that hot July afternoon, about 70 clinicians sat stuffed into the non-air-conditioned room to listen to me. My fears of ridicule, if not outright attack, were not realized. Instead, participants were engaged, supportive, curious, and quite moved by the model and case. Many encouraged me to publish the information, which led to my first article on this subject in the *Transactional Analysis Journal* in 2018.

Colleagues back home continued to suggest I publish a book about the model, but I declined for a long time out of fear of professional criticism, focusing instead on publishing journal articles that only hinted at how the model continued to expand.

My decision to publish the expanded model in this book, which includes forms of physical interaction that I have termed *body analysis*, was motivated by continued collegial encouragement and my belief in the importance of this type of treatment for people who have suffered all types of embodied trauma. For many such individuals, their trauma issues require treatment that addresses their experience not only through talk but also through touch. This is what I have been able to create for many of my patients, and it is the purpose of this book: to introduce a comprehensive model of how physical engagement with trauma patients can become a standard practice in some forms of embodied trauma therapy.

Review of Ongoing Terms in the Book

For those readers who may be unfamiliar with certain therapeutic terms, I will briefly describe a few here that I use throughout the book.

Ego state and *self-state* are terms from transactional analysis and psychoanalysis respectively. In my training in transactional analysis, there was an emphasis on recognizing and working directly with the three main ego states: Parent, Adult, and Child. In contemporary psychoanalysis, the comparable term is self-state. Both of these constructs are used to define when a person is in a state that contains thoughts, feelings, and/or behaviors from a certain moment in their past, such as the feelings and sensations of remembering a pleasant day or traumatic experience in childhood. These states can become activated during an event or circumstance in present-day life that seems similar to a past experience. For example, an adult whose family moved to a new country when they were 7 years old may, as an adult, reexperience the fears and loneliness from that period when starting college, beginning a new job, or moving to a new apartment or home. Often the work in both transactional analysis and psychoanalysis focuses on recognizing and exploring specific ego states or self-states of the patient.

These terms are used to help symbolize experienced phenomena and are not actual entities. When we speak of an ego state or self-state we are attempting to create a frame for an experience in order to be able to think about, observe, and make contact with it. In addition, these constructs are not suggestive of a multiple personality. Rather, they are ways of describing thoughts, feelings, and sensations that seem anchored in past experiences.

Ego states and self-states can also be applied to physical sensations and used in work with touch in ways that are similar to how they are used in talk therapy. The terms ego state or self-state can be used in processing and symbolizing embodied experiences that become more integrated into the patient's sense of self. A patient can revisit specific physical events and sensations from the past that had been either traumatic (e.g., physical abuse) or unavailable (e.g., comforting touch) within specific ego states or self-states. These processes can then be experienced in the patient's adult body, and the person can discover the return of a bodily capacity to do something(s) in the here and now with a trusted other. Body experiences from different ages, symbolized as a child ego state or self-state, can be integrated and transformed through therapeutic physical contact.

I also make use of several terms to describe the physical interactions of patient and therapist within therapy. These include *embodied therapy, body psychotherapy, touch, physical contact*, and *physical engagement*. I use them because body-to-body contact in treatment is complex and expansive, and I want to use words that symbolize this expansiveness rather than reducing it to just generic "touch." In addition, the term body psychotherapy is generally used when I am referring to traditional body psychotherapies in which the focus is primarily on the patient's body with limited integration of psychoanalytic psychotherapy.

The reader will find I generally use the terms *psychoanalytic psychotherapy* and *therapy* to reference multiple types of therapy. I also use the term *therapist* for the provider of this treatment. I use these terms to create the inclusiveness I believe is part of embodied therapy. That is, with training in some form of mental health therapy and then training in embodied therapy, clinicians of different disciplines can effectively use embodied therapy with patients. When speaking of my own work with patients, I often use the term *psychoanalysis* because I am a certified psychoanalyst and work analytically with my patients.

Research and References

In this book, I have not cited every theory that has influenced my work and this model. These include research in neuroscience, attachment theory, body-centered approaches, trauma research, transactional analysis, and psychoanalysis. This decision was based on my wish that the book remains primarily focused on the clinical side of embodied therapy. In addition, research and theory are interwoven in this model, and attempting to attribute one type of either to certain parts of the model would not be reflective of the expansive use of research and theory. However, for readers who are interested, I have detailed research, theory, and the authors who influenced this model in some of my previous publications (Novak, 2008, 2013, 2016, 2018, 2021).

References

Bacal, H. A. (2011). The power of specificity in psychotherapy: When therapy works and when it doesn't. Jason Aronson.

Novak, E. T. (2008). Integrating neurobiological findings with transactional analysis in trauma work: Linking "there and then" self states with "here and now" ego states. *Transactional Analysis Journal*, 38, 303–319. doi:10.1177/036215370803800405.

Novak, E. T. (2013). Combining traditional ego state theory and relational approaches to transactional analysis in working with trauma and dissociation. *Transactional Analysis Journal*, 43(3), 186–196. doi:10.1177/0362153713509952.

Novak, E. T. (2016). When transgressing standard therapeutic frames leads to progressive change, not ethical violations: Secret garden work. *Transactional Analysis Journal*, 48(1), 18–32. doi:10.1080/03621537.2018.1397962.

Novak, E. T. (2017, 27 July). *Touching trauma without violating boundaries: Using informed physical contact to integrate traumatized ego states* [*Workshop*]. World Transactional Analysis Conference, Berlin, Germany.

Novak, E. T. (2018). A model of informed physical contact in psychotherapy. *Transactional Analysis Journal*, 48(1), 18–32. doi:10.1080/03621537.2018.1397962.

Novak, E. T. (2021). Working in the terrain of the damaged self core. *Transactional Analysis Journal*, 51(3), 241–253. doi:10.1080/03621537.2021.1950968.

Chapter 1

Stolen Bodies and Sacred Spaces

Almost everyone who endures some form of bodily abuse or neglect, crippling physical injury, or medical illness has had their body or parts of their embodied experience stolen from them. This creates conflictual relationships with their own bodies as well as in relation to others. The stolen embodied experiences will vary in degree and manifest in ways that are particular to each person. Although sometimes obvious, more often such embodied thefts remain hidden not only from others but often even from the person.

In my psychoanalytic training, I began to notice similarities between trauma theories that addressed ways patients defend against cognitive memories of trauma and ways they defend against connecting body sensations to such trauma. As is well known in trauma theory, the body often becomes split off from the mind during a traumatic event. For people who have been abused, the body often becomes viewed as parts—some good, some bad, some disgusting—with even some parts or sensations totally ignored or put out of awareness.

Such a fragmented body holds the memory and meaning of the trauma, and it may become reintegrated if the person can find someone, usually a skilled therapist, who can help them recognize and reclaim their body. This is long-term work and requires developing a trusting relationship between patient and therapist along with the return of the person's ability to be curious about their own body. Often patients are not even aware of how limited their relationship with their own bodies has become or the ways they avoid physical contact.

Some traumatized individuals adjust by creating a relationship with their body that may look healthy but conceals internal disgust, contempt, and shame of their body. They may engage in daily workouts, be fit and toned, dress for success, and present an external body confidence that hides a very different internal body perception. Others relate to their body as if it were a tool, instrument, or as Williams (2021) notes, "a survival machine" (p. 39). They ignore pain and other body warnings and push their body beyond healthy physical limits, often causing muscle or nerve damage requiring

DOI: 10.4324/9781003215745-2

medical attention that they also ignore. Still others deal with their disdain and hatred for their body by abusing or ignoring it altogether. Such individuals wreck their physical well-being through poor nutrition, limited physical exercise, drugs and alcohol, and dismissing, if not exacerbating, health issues. They experience their body as weak, disgusting, inert, and unable to be used in healthy and enjoyable ways. In many such cases, serious health issues are ignored even following empathic confrontations and attempted interventions from concerned loved ones.

Sadly, many victims of bodily abuse have given up on bodily pleasure. From the warm embrace of a friend or family member, to sensual and sexual pleasures, the enjoyment of the physical body has been ravaged and replaced with embodied trauma flashbacks that seem indiscriminately activated even when engaging in healthy forms of physical contact. This leads to feelings of terror and shame. Relief after a sexual experience without an embodied flashback is seen as success, whereas the possibility of intense embodied pleasure, even orgasm, has been given up as impossible or no longer desired. This is to avoid disappointment and embodied flashbacks that bring into consciousness ways their trauma continues to intrude on their body.

In embodied therapy, these ingrained embodied limitations can become understood, treated, and transformed to various degrees, leading to a return of the capacity to enjoy bodily pleasure. Such therapy also helps to address issues of chronic anxiety and depression that originate within embodied trauma flashbacks or a more subtle embodied memory that is not yet being linked to the patient's mood or emotions. This is often seen in feelings of chronic loneliness, depression, or anxiety due to early childhood neglect. In many instances, the patient feels emotions and sensations that are connected to insufficient physical holding or attachment. Without therapy to help the patient recognize this link and then find ways to physically address those issues, the person will likely continue to suffer. Adding a theory of embodied therapy to psychotherapy and psychoanalysis creates a more comprehensive treatment for certain trauma patients.

Sacred Spaces in Embodied Treatment

"Sacred" is a word usually associated with religion, but it also offers an apt image of the type of office space and therapeutic relationship required to work within the private world of a stolen body. Perhaps *therapeutic reverence* may carry a less religious overtone for such a process. The therapist's deep respect and commitment in relating to a patient who had their body stolen is essential for working in the terrain of embodied trauma.

For many people with embodied trauma, some form of physical engagement with a trained professional is a necessity. At the same time, the idea of working with touch in therapy, even with a knowledgeable and trusted therapist, can be an anxiety-filled proposition. For patients who have abuse histories, many forms of physical engagement are viewed with suspicion. This is one of many reasons why moving into physical contact with a patient needs to occur after months, if not years, of working to create the type of space and therapeutic relationship that can provide a feeling of safety, especially when embodied trauma flashbacks occur.

Creating this sacred space begins in talk therapy. In psychoanalytic psychotherapy without touch, a similar space and relationship are required for the patient to feel safe in disclosing parts of themselves that they keep hidden from the world. Maurice Apprey has taught me to enter into this hidden world of the patient with the recognition that the therapist is the most important person this part of the patient's self has ever met. This way of thinking is not about some form of therapeutic grandiosity. Rather, it speaks to the type of relational experience in a therapeutic setting that matches the parts of the patient's self that are becoming available in treatment. As the work with the patient's trauma progresses, the relational space Apprey speaks of continues to deepen. The patient becomes more trusting of the therapist and moves into the brutal but necessary work of talking about the details of their trauma and feeling the kaleidoscope of emotions and body sensations associated with it. The quality of the therapist's empathic presence and their ability to remain present in these intense and often unbearable feelings determines whether it is appropriate to include embodied therapy in treatment. The talk therapy also functions as a therapeutic frame and template for work in the initial stages of embodied therapy. The patient and therapist can return to specific details already addressed in talk therapy and now focus directly on the patient's somatic sensations linked to them.

Another important embodied dynamic in creating this sacred space is for the patient's body to be seen and related to as subject rather than object, with the therapist's body being an object to be made use of by the patient. Since most forms of physical abuse result in an objectification of the abused person's body, it is essential to create a relational space in which the patient does not feel objectified or used by the therapist to gratify their own needs. The ability of the patient to reclaim a sense of their body as subject rather than object is one of the more transformational outcomes of embodied therapy. This is only possible when the patient and therapist can create a safe and sacred space that facilitates the level of trust necessary for embodied therapy.

Why Does a Patient Need to Be Touched in Therapy

Therapists often ask me why patients cannot just do bodywork with their significant other. If the patient is in a relationship in which they can receive touch, why does the therapist need to provide it in embodied therapy? I answer the question in two parts. First, a patient's significant other can also talk to them about their trauma issues, so why do they need to be in psychoanalysis or psychotherapy to talk about their trauma? This question leads into the second part: Like most other dynamics in therapy, touch between patient and therapist carries different motivations, meanings, and possibilities that are not available in any other relationship.

For example, a patient who was physically or sexually abused as a child certainly could experience touch with their therapist as uncomfortable and anxiety provoking and may therefore prefer a therapeutic relationship with no touch. In fact, it is usually important early in treatment to avoid physical contact until the therapist has an in-depth understanding of the patient and their issues and until the patient experiences the therapeutic relationship and frame as safe and predictable.

Over the course of treatment, however, the absence of physical contact also forecloses opportunities to work more directly with the patient's embodied sensations as evoked by direct physical contact. Experiences of safe and informed touch in therapy can help patients become more curious about when and why specific forms of physical engagement create anxiety or embodied trauma flashbacks and to work with and through these sensations. In this way, touch provides a unique opportunity for patients to explore their traumatized self-states in ways that other relationships, including with a significant other, cannot provide. Including touch in therapy connects the therapeutic relationship directly with the patient's conflicts around touch. The therapist can help the patient explore their fears, avoidance, enjoyment, and desire for physical connections. In addition, the patient can often revisit trauma memories with more curiosity and depth while being physically anchored in their physical connection with the therapist.

Although it may be possible for patients to address embodied issues in the context of a personal relationship, I do not believe doing so is in the best interests of the relationship, given the intensity and relational dynamics of embodied trauma. Issues such as transference, countertransference, enactments, and reenactments that occur in talk therapy are also a part of embodied therapy. These issues and listening to and absorbing the explicit details of a partner's abuse history may be beyond what is healthy for the relationship and may instead be best addressed with a therapist.

Within a psychoanalytic frame, Bollas (2013) addressed people working with their partner on their emotions related to disturbing childhood events. He wrote about it in ways that can also be applied to embodied therapy: "the child that is stunned by a disturbing event in reality has an unconscious sense, or preconception, that someday they will be able to turn to an empathic other in order to make sense of the experience" (p. 71). Bollas suggested that often this empathic other is realized through a relationship with a lover.

> Owing to the promise of love and the intoxicating feeling of this relationship, it is not unusual for the self to realize stored self-states in the form of powerful disclosures to the lover. The problem is that, although

the lover may feel gratified and privileged initially to be gifted such precious secrets, it may not be long before they feel disturbed by it and are unsure what to do. It is not enough for their partner to have "got it off their chest" as there has been no abreaction of the affect buried in the event. It needs to be experienced in the presence of an other, who will transform it into meaning. This is ordinarily far too much for the lover to do—although many try—and the stress of the situation can prove too much for the couple, who may even break up under the strain.

(pp. 71–72)

If we take Bollas's ideas and apply them to embodied trauma, we see important similarities. I believe a child or adult who was the victim of physical trauma has a preconception or hope that someday they will find an understanding and empathic other who can be with them in relation to their embodied trauma, help them transform their experience, and heal. Often these forms of trauma only become available to cognitive memory when a trusted other has become a part of the person's life.

Bollas's ideas around what a partner can handle and what is probably beyond their abilities applies to embodied issues and flashbacks as well. For a partner to be able to stay with embodied flashbacks and transform them into meaning, especially when their own touch is what activated the flashback, is an unrealistic expectation and can also result in strain that can lead to a breakup.

A therapist, on the other hand, can attend to embodied issues and flashbacks in ways a patient's significant other cannot. The therapist can process with the patient the feelings that physical interactions may evoke, such as love, hate, self-disgust or repulsion, longing, relief, pleasure, fear, and hope. They can do that in ways that are similar to how issues of transference, countertransference, projection, enactments, and other experiences in psychoanalytic psychotherapy are processed.

Informed and disciplined touch moves the patient and therapist more directly into the bodily experience of trauma memories where they can be recognized, physically felt, and analyzed. In this way, new experiences of touch can provide opportunities for patients to experience touch in fundamentally new ways both relationally and intrapsychically.

When using touch to address certain self-state experiences, physical contact can serve an integrative function that is not available in most relationships. A patient can revisit specific physical processes from the past that had been either traumatic (e.g., physical abuse) or unavailable (e.g., reparative touch). These can then be experienced in the patient's adult body so they can discover the return of a bodily capacity to do some thing(s) in the here and now with a trusted other. Body experiences from different ages and self-states can then be integrated through a combination of engaging in physical contact and processing the experie

I Don't Touch Patients ... but Actually I Do

Although there is increasing awareness in contemporary psychoanalytic psychotherapy of the importance of the embodied experience of both the patient and the therapist, most theories of treatment continue to exclude or marginalize the option of direct physical contact. The profession continues to struggle because of the early edict of "no touch" that began in psychoanalytic theory (Mintz, 1969). The complicated history between psychoanalysis and the physical body has cast suspicion on touch, reducing it to, at best, a provisional act and, at worst, some form of boundary violation. Touch has often been viewed as acting out, need gratification, sexual transference, or even sexual countertransference on the part of the therapist. From a clinical standpoint, these perceptions make the possibility of therapeutic touch difficult to consider and have often led to a privileging of mind over body, even in embodied trauma work.

When I discuss my model of therapy with colleagues, usually I hear initially that they do not work with embodied therapy. Yet almost inevitably, as we talk, they mention a handshake, a hug, or even holding a patient's hand in session. They describe the situation that created the possibility of touch and why that form of physical engagement seemed important. Perhaps my initial discussion about using touch provides an opportunity or welcoming space in which they feel comfortable speaking about their own physical connections with patients. These exchanges affirm what I already suspected: Many therapists, psychologists, psychotherapists, psychoanalysts, and other mental health professionals do engage in physical contact with some patients, and only those who adhere to the strictest rules of no touch consider an occasional handshake or hug out of bounds. And yet seldom are these forms of contact explored in any meaningful way. In addition, the anxiety, secrecy, or uncertainty expressed when discussing their use of touch indicates that the shift to embodied therapy is not seen or treated as a form of therapy. Rather, physical contact is viewed as a less than optimal, spontaneous add-on at specific moments in talk therapy rather than being a form of treatment.

The professional suspicion and dismissal, if not contempt, for the use of therapeutic physical contact in psychoanalytic psychotherapy perpetuates a mind–body split. The fact that many therapists do engage in some form of physical contact with certain patients is another reason why we need to establish theoretical and clinical models of embodied therapy within therapeutic professions.

To Touch or Not Touch: A Therapeutic Decision

In psychoanalysis and psychotherapy, the decision about whether to include touch in treatment is usually assumed to be the therapist's, often influenced by professional suspicion and limited support for such work. This pulls decisions around touch out of the patient–therapist dyad and into a more professional realm that limits patient input.

In my own attempts to find an analyst who would use physical contact as part of my work on my childhood traumas, I often heard some form of "I don't touch my patients." Sometimes I wondered, but never asked, why then we shook hands as I entered the consultation room. When I did inquire about the reasons for a no-touch policy, I usually heard a scripted, dogmatic response about touch being confusing, a corrective experience, and an unnecessary and/or dismissive response when I explained my own ideas and experiences about how and why touch would be a beneficial part of my work. Already in the initial consultation, the foreclosure of even the possibility of touch created unforeseen issues and conflicts for me that would be played out in multiple ways if we decided to work together. I know that these issues and conflicts were not unique to me, and I will discuss three of them briefly here.

First, by framing "no touch" within a policy or rule forecloses opportunities for the patient and therapist to explore together the therapeutic risks and benefits of touch in treatment. This makes it even harder for a trauma patient to initiate and discuss this already difficult topic. Fears of being seen as "creepy" or "perverse" often inhibit a patient from talking about wanting some form of touch even when it is available. This can also be the case with something like massage. Because of their fears, it is still difficult, especially for trauma patients, to request a type of touch that would be appropriate, such as lighter touch or spending more time on a specific area of the body.

Initiating a conversation with a therapist about possible touch, including something like a hug at the end of a session, when there is a strong position against it is a daunting task for patients with trauma histories and issues around physical contact. They fear being seen as manipulative or seductive and often believe that they are not entitled to any form of embodied relief or comfort. Even in my own practice, despite knowing that I am open to physical contact, many patients with trauma histories have difficulty requesting it.

On the other hand, having a rule or policy in place can be a relief to trauma patients and provide them with a safe space in which to speak about their traumas because they know there will be no physical contact. However, such a stance also deprives patients of exploring and making decisions within the therapeutic relationship. By incorporating decisions about touch into the therapeutic structure, even a no-touch agreement becomes part of the working relationship rather than something decided exclusively by the therapist. I have had patients with abuse histories say they would never work with touch and that I would never touch them. That was an important moment in their therapy because they were able to use their own voice and set their own no-touch boundary. The therapist's acceptance and respect in such cases can be an important therapeutic moment for someone who has been abused.

Second, a no-touch rule or policy creates a hard physical boundary that may create complications if touch ever does occur in the relationship. A handshake or hug after an intense session or an embrace before a long break may feel suspicious given the patient and therapist have now "broken" a rule. Any comfort the patient might feel from it may be negated by a sense that maybe they manipulated or seduced the therapist or that they themselves were seduced. A softer boundary, with an openness to touch if it is ever merited, avoids this situation—one that I have often heard about in consultation with other therapists. A softer boundary keeps open the possibility of touch and makes it easier for a patient to disclose when a certain issue or experience in the session evokes the desire for touch.

A third issue with a no-touch rule is that trauma experiences that create mind and body splits are now re-created within the therapeutic encounter (S. Kiersky, personal communication, 13 April 2020). I suspect that many patients experience, but may not be able to verbalize, that a no-touch policy is received by traumatized self-states as an indication that their analyst is afraid to touch them. The split between mind and body confirms their belief that there is something wrong with their body or touch. McLaughlin (2000) said this about his own aversion to and withholding of touch with some patients who wanted it: "[My refusal] … confirmed their worst fears and led to a protracted and stalemated analysis that the two of us could neither resolve nor get beyond" (p. 68).

To reduce issues like these, I often introduce my openness to embodied therapy early in my work with trauma patients. I briefly talk about the importance of attending to body issues in such work, and these early discussions include some attention to the patient's perceptions of and relationship to their body. The patient's level of comfort in speaking about their body can provide valuable information that we will make use of throughout their analysis. I also believe these initial conversations signal to patients that I am open to and comfortable with addressing the body and body issues in a curious and respectful manner that will not feel intrusive. In this way, the person can start to become more curious about their body right from the start of treatment. The patient also hears my belief that they have a legitimate right to be touched, whether or not this occurs in our work. I also let patients know that I work with body processes both with and without touch and that work with touch generally does not occur until later in treatment. I want to reduce any worries the patient might have that I expect touch to be part of the work.

One of the reasons I believe it is important to address the issue of possible touch early on is that most patients have heard and believe that touch in therapy is not allowed. When a patient learns that I sometimes do embodied therapy, they invariably say something like, "I didn't know you were allowed to do that." So, an ongoing education process about what work with touch does and does not look like is important as we consider whether or not including touch in treatment would be therapeutic for them. Including the possibility of physical engagement in treatment can create both curiosity and apprehension, which can be explored in ways that allow the patient to gain insight into their embodied issues even if touch never occurs.

I often hear, and have also said, that touch with certain patients may be ill advised because it can create more confusion and anxiety for them, especially early in treatment. The traditional therapeutic frame that includes a solid boundary between the patient's and therapist's bodies provides space for patients to explore their traumas without the confusion of touch in the work. For many individuals, this is enough and all that they want in treatment. However, I think we do not talk enough about patients' confusion or thoughts about us *not* touching them. As I said earlier, many patients find that talking about touch in a traditional, no-physical-contact relationship is difficult to initiate, so often such discussions must be initiated by the therapist.

The embodied therapy that I outline in this book is for patients who want to experience more once they begin to understand that more is even possible via forms of embodied therapy. If psychoanalytic psychotherapy does not include embodied therapy, then the patient needs to understand that they are up against a therapeutic limit rather than the limits of what they can accomplish relative to their trauma and their body.

The Processing of Touch

A key component in any form of physical contact between patient and therapist is the ability to talk about the patient's experience of the interaction. This can range from exploring a specific sensation to a more detailed processing of multiple sensations. Within the processing, the therapist assists the patient in exploring meanings, associations, and other thoughts and feelings about their experience of the touch. Often a certain type of touch will bring to the surface issues that have been avoided, split off, or may have been unconscious. The processing of the physical interactions helps to symbolize and create meaning around these new forms of therapeutic touch, which is fundamentally different from their abuse.

This processing can also be used with bodywork that occurs outside of the therapy within a modality such as massage. A patient may have important embodied experiences while receiving a massage. However, unless these experiences are symbolized and processed, they are less likely to be integrated and linked to specific self-states. Often processing helps anchor this new experience within the patient's mind and body, thereby creating a form of mastery over a trauma.

Processing even supposedly simple physical interactions can uncover a multitude of thoughts, feelings, and associations. Something as basic as a handshake after a session can create many opportunities for exploration and curiosity. Who initiated the handshake? How did it occur? What part of the session work did the handshake seem most connected to? What motivated the handshake? Did it feel like a one-time event or will it occur again? What was the quality of eye contact? What were the facial expressions? Was it a firm or soft handshake, long or short? Was the pressure between the hands congruent or incongruent? Would the patient have preferred a hug, and if so, why did they initiate a handshake instead? All these and even more questions can arise from what might seem like a simple form of touch.

Touching the Third Rail: The Integration of Embodied Therapy and Psychoanalysis

For years I was unaware of how I was working within a body and mind split in my clinical work with patients. I was also not aware that combining embodied therapy and psychoanalytic psychotherapy was even possible because of how I had experienced bodywork in the first decade of my therapeutic career. My personal embodied work took place in weekend workshops separated from my psychotherapy, which occurred in weekly individual sessions without touch.

In addition, the body techniques, reading, and consultations I was engaged in all were heavily focused on the *patient*'s body and their responses to the work, with limited, if any, processing of the therapist's body and reactions to the work. From a psychoanalytic perspective, the emphasis was on the patient's transference without much consideration of the therapist's countertransference. I now understand that part of the reason for the absence of curiosity around countertransference had to do with how body psychotherapy was being conducted. The therapist's job was to watch and work with the patient's body in ways that resembled a more traditional one-person psychotherapy. For many years in working with touch, I followed this model, which, in essence, separated both body from mind and patient from therapist. In fact, the idea of an integration of embodied therapy and psychotherapy along with working in a two-person embodied relational field did not occur to me until I began my own psychoanalytic training.

In psychoanalytic training, the analysand is required to undergo their own analysis, which is one of the most important components of the process. When I was in my training analysis, I was also involved in my own bodywork, which, in retrospect, became an adjunct to my training analysis. In working simultaneously with both psychoanalysis and embodied therapy, I was surprised to discover that almost everything that I was experiencing in my analysis I was also experiencing in my bodywork. The split between mind and body was still there because the two forms of therapy were conducted by different professionals. A significant shift occurred when I was able to take my embodied work back to my analyst, who was able to help me process it and explore the relational dynamics between my massage therapist and me. I then took that processing back to my massage therapist and we began to understand how to make more use of the relational field between us within the context of my transference and her countertransference.

I was incredibly fortunate in my training analysis to work with an analyst who viewed my bodywork as enhancing my analysis rather than detracting from it. She remained open to that framework throughout my analysis, and her insights in processing my embodied therapy were a crucial part of that work. I was also fortunate to work with a massotherapist who was willing to engage in embodied therapy with my traumas, including processing the massage sessions with me. That is often considered inappropriate in massage because transference and countertransference are viewed critically.

I encountered that view in my own brief massage training. One of the books used in class (Beck, 2010) addressed the issues of transference and countertransference in ways that were outdated but still taught in massage training. Beck referred to transference as involving "misperceptions that the client might have toward the practitioner or therapist" (p. 42) and that "Transference usually tends to diminish the effectiveness of the therapeutic relationship" (p. 42). Relative to countertransference, Beck wrote that "It is usually unconscious and always detrimental to the therapeutic process" (p. 43). In a disturbing paragraph, he even blames the client for the therapist's countertransference: "Many times a client's transference, when unrecognized, will spawn countertransference on the part of the unwitting practitioner. This is nearly always a recipe for disappointment and possible disaster for the practitioner" (p. 43). With such dire and misinformed warnings, how can a massage therapist feel comfortable processing the client's thoughts and feelings evoked during a massage?

The experience of transference and countertransference as dangerous has not been my experience in massage or what I have heard when massage therapists speak of their professional relationship with clients. The aversion to recognizing transference and countertransference as a natural part of the relationship creates a body/mind split in massage that needs to be addressed and reevaluated by the profession. In contemporary psychoanalysis, we are trained that transference and countertransference are informative, not sources of seduction. It is the same in bodywork. Touch is an ongoing communication used to inform the process of embodied transformation. By educating not only massage therapists but other helping professionals who work directly with the body, issues such as transference and countertransference can be recognized as important components of the therapeutic process and addressed rather than avoided. My model of embodied therapy can be used to help professionals in all forms of bodywork understand how to deal with the more psychological aspects of it, including transference and countertransference.

My own analytic training, which focused on integrating my experiences in analysis and massage therapy, helped me begin to consider the ways I could start to integrate embodied therapy and psychoanalytic psychotherapy in my practice. This also coincided with my increased ability to work with patients in a more two-person relational way, which allowed me to use both one-person and two-person approaches as needed. Over many years, I became more comfortable and confident in integrating embodied therapy and psychoanalysis, understanding when and at what depth this integration was possible and useful with specific patients.

I have referred to this integration of embodied therapy and psychoanalysis metaphorically as "touching the third rail." On many electric trains, the third rail carries the high electric charge essential for making the system work. However, that rail can be fatal if touched. In therapy, there is a level of intensity when the "rails" of psychoanalysis and embodied therapy are combined into a "third rail." However, rather than causing injury or death, in my work with certain patients, this combination has facilitated transformations at embodied and psychic levels that have been beyond anything that they or I could have imagined. Their ability to reclaim their stolen body and relate differently to their body and the bodies of others has been remarkable.

Nonetheless, working in this way does have inherent risks, as is the case with all forms of treatment. And success is not guaranteed. My model of embodied therapy takes into account that each therapeutic relationship uses embodied therapy in different ways and depths. This is another reason why a continuum of touch is built into the model as described in Chapter 2.

I suspect most clinicians who read this book and choose to pursue working with specific patients in embodied therapy will not engage in a full integration of embodied therapy and psychoanalytic psychotherapy. There are not many patients who are able to experience this form of long-term treatment, even with me. The intensity of the work, the level of commitment required from both therapist and patient, and the depth of trust needed means such therapy usually takes years. However, sometimes the work can be designed to include some moments of this form of integration and can be conducted primarily within a separation of these two forms of therapy. The embodied therapy may also be carried out using a more one-person modality, and therapists may also use brief embodied therapy as detailed in Chapter 5.

Alternatively, therapists might find that they or their patients prefer that embodied therapy be conducted outside of their psychoanalytic psychotherapy. The patient can then bring their embodied work back to the therapy for processing. As described earlier and also in Chapter 3, this was the form my own bodywork took following my first therapy and one I often still use with patients. The patient's embodied work can take on multiple forms, such as massage, yoga, athletics, and types of dance. Even in these instances, the model presented in this book provides ways of thinking about the body and physical contact that can be used in the processing of these transformative forms of embodied work.

References

Beck, M. F. (2010). *Theory and practice of therapeutic massage* (5th ed.). Milady Publishing.

Bollas, C. (2013). *Catch them before they fall: The psychoanalysis of breakdown*. Routledge. https://doi.org/10.4324/9780203069547.

McLaughlin, J. T. (2000). The problem and place of physical contact in analytic work: Some reflections on handholding in the analytic situation. *Psychoanalytic Inquiry, 209(1)*, 65–81. https://doi.org/10.1080/07351692009348875.

Mintz, E. E. (1969). Touch and the psychoanalytic tradition. *Psychoanalytic Review, 56(3)*, 365–376. https://doi.org/10.1037/h0088759.

Williams, P. (2021). *The authority of tenderness: The dignity and the true self in psychoanalysis.* Routledge. DOI:10.4324/9781003176862-7.

Chapter 2

A Model of Informed Physical Contact

Since I first published this model in 2018, it has undergone several revisions and expanded to include more ways of using physical engagement in treatment. The model provides a systematic process for embodied therapy whereby theory and clinical experience are used to inform the depth, pace, and intensity of the work. This model is the cumulation of my 30+ years of study and experience with body psychotherapy, transactional analysis, and psychoanalysis, including my own intense bodywork on my trauma issues. The model also incorporates the expanding research on trauma and dissociation, which continues to highlight the importance of working with the physical body in treatment as discussed in Chapter 1. Integrating body psychotherapy, trauma research and theory, and psychoanalytic psychotherapy into one model has provided many of my patients the opportunity to address both mind and body in the context of therapy to deal with their trauma.

Addressing both mind and body in one treatment model creates a more expansive relationship between patient and therapist, one in which the patient can feel known in thought, emotions, and physical experience. As stated in Chapter 1, informed and disciplined touch moves patients more directly into embodied trauma memories where such memories can be observed, analyzed, and physically felt. This creates opportunities for the patient to explore and transform their embodied trauma memories.

In my model, physical contact can also serve an integrative function for specific traumatized self-states. A patient can revisit situations from the past that were either traumatic (e.g., physical abuse) or lacking in needed physical connection (e.g., comforting touch). In treatment, situations that typically activate embodied flashbacks can be safely revisited in the here and now with a trusted therapist. Through the embodied connection with their therapist, the patient can explore and discover the return of a bodily capacity to do something(s) that attends to these embodied trauma memories in the here and now. In this work, traumatic body experiences from different ages and self-states are transformed and integrated into the patient's adult body in fundamentally new ways.

A model of embodied therapy can also provide neurological benefits. Eldredge and Cole (2007), referencing the work of Fonagy et al. (2002),

DOI: 10.4324/9781003215745-3

suggested that caregivers need to help children manage and regulate their affective states because a child's immature nervous system cannot yet regulate intense affect independently. They wrote, "The caregiver in a sense lends her mature nervous system to assist the child to develop the capacity for self-regulation" (pp. 83–84). In psychoanalytic psychotherapy, in the context of the emotional intensity of revisiting trauma memories, a patient may make use of their therapist in a similar way.

A significant component of my model is the processing of the patient's thoughts and feelings about physical contact. In addition to more overt processing (e.g., what felt safe, confusing, more helpful, less helpful), time can be spent exploring ways of languaging the somatic sensations that were evoked and are available to the patient. The processing of somatic sensations is similar to the way dreams are processed in contemporary therapies through exploring associations, fantasies, multiple meanings, transference, and creating links.

Another important component of my model is the continuum of touch. The model moves from basic and more social forms of touch (e.g., handshakes) into more intense, complex forms of physical engagement that require even more study and clinical experience. The model also provides the patient and therapist with a framework that can be used to assess what type of touch might best address the patient's issues. The therapist can use these categories of touch to help assess when certain forms of embodied therapy are beyond their abilities, those of the patient, or what is needed in the treatment. This model is used and referred to throughout this book and applied to the cases presented.

All Touch Is Not Equal: Categories of Touch

Touch in the therapeutic encounter, as in life outside the office, has many different meanings and motivations. In an earlier version of this model (Novak, 2018), I identified four categories of touch that help to contextualize physical contact in treatment and provide a framework for physical contact. Since that writing, my understanding and skills in working with touch and body processes have expanded to include a fifth category, which I call *body analysis.*

My specific emphasis has been on categories that match the clinical process of working with physical contact with patients whose relationship with their bodies has suffered as a result of embodied trauma. The way a clinician makes use of these categories to develop a working frame in their practice may be more important than the actual ways certain types of touch and bodywork are categorized.

The five categories I use range on a continuum from more superficial or social touch to complicated and complex forms of working with touch and body processes in body analysis. On this continuum, patient and therapist have structured treatment options that can be used to address symptom relief or engage in deeper, longer term work with an emphasis on embodied transformation. Thus, this model provides the therapist with a systematic approach to embodied therapy.

The five categories are: pass-bys (W. Cornell, personal communication, 6 September 2012), completion touch, containing-informing touch, somatic mastery and modulation (Klopstech, 2009), and body analysis. Within these five categories, the experience of touch moves from structured approaches to more spontaneous forms of embodied work as the patient and therapist become more in tune with one another and the patient's therapeutic needs. Metaphorically speaking, the categories in this model begin as a form of ballroom dancing and end in a form of tango.

One of the benefits of having a five-category model of touch is that the initial work can begin within a heavily structured and tightly contained frame in which physical engagements are limited to specific forms of touch that are planned out beforehand and processed during and after the work. From this heavily structured starting point, the patient and therapist can then assess the viability of moving the work into other categories, if and as appropriate.

A common concern in the use of therapeutic touch is that the patient may experience or interpret therapeutic physical contact differently than intended by the therapist. These concerns are reduced when the therapist makes use of this model because the physical interactions can remain within a particular category and only move into other categories on the continuum if both patient and therapist feel comfortable and there is a clear therapeutic benefit. In addition, working through the full continuum usually takes years. By the time embodied treatment moves into the final category of body analysis, the patient and therapist will have an expansive understanding and trust of both the work and one another.

It should be noted that these five flexible categories have significant overlap because touch can evoke and create different experiences and meanings at various phases of treatment. I will briefly define and describe the five categories here and subsequently refer to them throughout the book and within the cases that are presented.

Pass-By Touch

Pass-bys are part of the social rituals or pleasantries exchanged on the way into or out of the office. These are probably the most common and superficial forms of touch (e.g., shaking hands, hand on shoulder, a quick hug), although they can often be "a rich source of information" (Holder, 2000, p. 50). These brief physical encounters are not even considered by some clinicians to come under a "no touch rule." For example, I often hear colleagues who say that they do not work with touch speak of engaging in such forms of touch with patients. Often a pass-by may be a reflexive act that occurs before any discussion about it. However, from an embodied therapy perspective, even these forms of touch may require some form of processing by the patient and therapist. This is especially true when a handshake or hug becomes a ritualized pass-by before or after many sessions. In such instances, the ritualized form of physical interaction can become problematic if the physical engagement is incongruent with the emotions of the session. An example of this would be a therapy in which each session begins or ends with a handshake. If during a session the patient experiences irritation or anger toward the therapist (or the therapist toward the patient), a handshake after the session may be at odds with what is occurring within the therapeutic relationship. In such instances, engaging in a ritualized pass-by may lead to dismissing the irritation or anger.

The initial greeting between patient and therapist in the office waiting room is the first opportunity for the therapist to experience and observe touch with a new patient in the form of a possible greeting handshake. My approach to this initial meeting has evolved over time, and although I rarely overtly initiate, I almost always engage in a handshake before or after a first session. In instances where we shake hands, I will internally process what I noticed and took from the exchange. This includes ways I may have implicitly contributed to inviting the interaction and what I noticed in the exchange. For example, was the handshake soft and friendly or firm and more formal? Was there eye contact? If so, did the patient seem comfortable or anxious making eye contact? These and other observations, such as facial expressions and body posture, can often be indicators of possible transference and countertransference dynamics in the early work in therapy.

Completion Touch

Panksepp (1998) used the phrase "contact comfort" (p. 271) to describe the neurological benefits of touch as studied in animals (e.g., the calming effect on baby chicks of being held). According to Panksepp, the benefit of contact comfort "is both obvious and poorly studied" (p. 272).

I have expanded on Panksepp's ideas about contact comfort to create a category that I term *completion touch*. This form of touch can be similar in behavior to a pass-by or some form of contact comfort (e.g., a hug or handshake), but with different meanings and slight differences in the way they are experienced. Generally, completion touch refers to the types of physical contact that occur after intense affective, emotional, or somatic memories connected to loss or trauma have surfaced in the session. Such touch creates a physical connection between the patient and therapist that integrates their physical bodies into what has occurred in the session. In this way, the touch "completes" the work because the patient and therapist experience connectedness not only in thought and feelings but also at a body level. Certainly, comfort can also be a part of this interaction for the patient.

In many instances, the advantage of this form of touch is that the physical contact often occurs after the patient and therapist have worked on and through a trauma flashback. Some patients may be unable to make use of touch when they are experiencing such a flashback. In addition, many therapists may be uncomfortable working with physical contact when a patient is feeling the emotions and somatic sensations of their trauma. Completion touch places physical connection outside of this reliving of feelings associated with trauma.

When trauma memories and flashbacks surface during a session, the process of grounding the patient near the end of the session is a central aspect of treatment. Completion touch may serve as a form of physical grounding that can help reduce any of the patient's internal disruptions that remain at the end of the session. Although empathic attunement may help the patient feel understood and metaphorically held, the patient may receive greater therapeutic benefits from an empathic physical connection. Within completion touch, the patient's embodied suffering is met with embodied empathy that also includes traces of contact comfort as described by Panksepp (1998). Used in this way, the physical connection functions as an important way of restabilizing and grounding the patient.

For many patients who experienced abusive touch in childhood, the repair from these forms of embodied traumas would have needed to include physical comfort, but that was not available or provided at the time. In therapy, a meaningful handshake, hug, or embrace at the end of the session can provided the patient with a here-and-now experience of this form of physical connection.

I have found patients who request this form of touch do so in an attempt to feel a human connection to the trusted person with whom they have just revealed their most private and painful experiences. The therapist's empathic handshake or embrace often is the difference between the patient leaving the office with a sense of internal peace or having to repair lingering intense emotions and body sensations for the next several hours on their own.

Completion touch is neither an attempt at a magical therapeutic shortcut or a therapeutic add-on. Rather, it can be an essential part of the reparative work with patients who are addressing their trauma histories.

In my private practice, it is not uncommon after an intense session of trauma work for a patient to hesitate as they make their way toward the door. The patient moves toward me rather than the door for a possible hug. In these instances, I almost never deny them the human connection of touch. However, if for some reason the requested form of touch is beyond what I am comfortable with that day, then I will make an adjustment. In the case of a hug that at that time does not feel quite right, I may offer a handshake instead. I own my therapeutic side of this decision saying that for some reason a handshake feels like a better ending for the day, and we can talk about this in our next session.

Many times, just knowing that some form of completion touch will be available if needed can make the revealing and reliving of trauma memories in session more tolerable for the patient.

Containing–Informing Touch

From the many therapists I have spoken with who have engaged in physical contact with patients, I believe that both pass-bys and completion touch are the most common forms of physical engagement between patient and therapist. These are generally less intimidating for both individuals than *containing–informing touch*, probably because the latter is generally more sustained and occurs during trauma work in session. In fact, containing–informing touch seems to mark the divide between brief touch encounters to sustained physical connection. It also marks the beginning of the shift from touch used after trauma work to touch used during work with trauma memories in session.

What is needed is for the patient and therapist to assess whether they think the patient can benefit from physical engagement when they are feeling embodied sensations from their trauma or if touch would be too disruptive or confusing in those moments. This is another example of how working via the continuum keeps the work informed, disciplined, and specific to the patient's needs. By the time this type of assessment is required, the patient and therapist will have already engaged in earlier categories of touch, which can help to inform this assessment.

Containing–informing touch also marks a movement into deeper intrapersonal and relational experiences that can call up multiple thoughts and feelings from within various self-states. This form of physical contact is used to both contain embodied sensations and provide information about how the patient experiences physical engagement with the therapist in these various self-states. Examples include the patient and therapist holding hands, sitting shoulder to shoulder, or the therapist placing their hand on the patient's shoulder or arm. As the work progresses, even placing an arm around one another might become a part of the work. These forms of touch create a physical anchor and also help patients begin to compare and contrast there-and-then trauma experiences with here-and-now therapeutic experiences with a trusted and physically attuned therapist.

Often in trauma therapy the work focuses on helping the patient develop ways of grounding themselves in order to reduce the intensity of an embodied flashback. Some patients express a strong desire to stay within what they are experiencing in order to discover more about their traumas and their bodily reactions. Unlike words or eye contact, which tend to interrupt the patient's immersion in their trauma memories, containing–informing touch provides a connection that helps the patient tolerate and stay within the intense trauma emotions and body sensations. The therapist's calming presence and physical availability helps the patient remain curious about what they are reexperiencing rather than pulling them out of the experience too soon. Instead of having to keep a part of themselves on watch for fear of becoming overwhelmed, the patient can focus more on their traumatized self-states, returning to the therapist's touch for grounding when needed. An example of this is the patient squeezing the therapist's hand when they begin to feel alone, anxious, or terrified in a trauma memory or embodied flashback. In these instances, containing–informing touch can be the difference between working within trauma memories or becoming overwhelmed by them.

The experience of containing–informing touch is similar to a parent going into their young child's bedroom just as the child is beginning to stir and gently touching or placing a hand on the child. Often, the child will take a deep breath and then fall back to sleep. When used therapeutically in this way, containing–informing touch can contribute to a patient's ability to stay in the moment and more fully observe and reflect on what is happening in their body.

As with completion touch, sometimes the possibility of touch is as important and effective with some patients as actual touch is with others. Knowing that their therapist is willing to touch them in ways that would help them contain embodied sensations during the session may be all the patient needs in order to trust moving deeper into their trauma memories.

For example, I had a patient whom I thought was feeling my attempts at connection with her without touch. I mentioned something reassuring about my taking her trauma seriously. After a brief internal reflection, I added, "But I would think you are over there saying to yourself, 'If Ed actually understood what was going on with me, he'd be over here sitting next to me holding my hand!'" She laughed and agreed, and this exchange helped opened up the possibility of touch if things became too intense for her. During her analysis, we did make use of physical contact three times. One occurred when I moved my chair closer to hers in order to hold hands during an intense retelling of a childhood trauma. The other two times involved a hug at the end of an intense session in which she had reexperienced trauma memories. Both hugs were initiated by her, and they moved beyond completion touch into containing–informing touch. She sobbed during these embraces in a way that had not been possible during the actual reexperiencing. She used our physical connection at the end of the session as a containing function for her intense expression of sadness over her traumas. In processing, I learned she would often spend 10 minutes crying after a session and that these hugs had helped her to cry with me instead of alone in her car.

Over time, containing–informing touch creates a connection within early self-states that leads to changes at both explicit and implicit levels of self-organization. In addition, the patient can relate to the therapist as a witness not only in thought (Stern, 2010) but also within the embodied experiences of the past. Containing–informing touch helps create a predictable, safe space in which traumatized self-states are addressed over multiple sessions. This new space is an important part of the embodied therapy frame if the work moves further along the continuum into somatic mastery and modulation and body analysis.

Somatic Mastery and Modulation

Somatic mastery and modulation (Klopstech, 2009) refers to forms of physical contact and work with body processes as they are used in traditional body-work and body psychotherapy. I have found these to be an important part of working with embodied trauma in psychoanalytic psychotherapy as well. This type of physical contact moves embodied therapy further along the touch continuum. Within this category, the primary focus is on increasing the patient's curiosity, understanding, and agency of their own body.

The development of classical body psychotherapy is generally attributed to Wilhelm Reich (1949), and most contemporary schools of body psychotherapy grew out of his work (Klopstech, 2009; Smith, 1985). Klopstech included in these diverse schools bioenergetic analysis (Lowen, 1975), radix (Kelley, 1978), formative psychology (Keleman, 1975), and biosynthesis (Boadella, 1987). Generally, these and many other forms of body psychotherapy require additional training or at least some personal work and experience in them.

Klopstech (2009) described these schools and clinical practices as centering

> on the 'energy body' of cells, muscles, flesh and movement, the observable body, the 'touch body', the body as experiencing and feeling agent in the present and the body as repository of history … the body represents freedom and impulse, … and what psychoanalysis labels as 'acting out' is labeled here as aliveness or vitality.
>
> (p. 16)

Klopstech (2009) also noted that in the body psychotherapies, "the body and not language, is at the heart of theory and treatment" (p. 16). The emphasis is on helping the patient create confidence and aliveness in their body personally and relationally, which is especially important in working with patients with a history of trauma. In such cases, there are several variations of techniques that can be used to address specific patient needs.

Smith (1985) distinguished between what he referred to as *soft techniques,* which include gentle interventions that allow for emotions and body awareness to emerge, and *hard techniques,* which are more forceful in design so as to release blocked energy and emotions. He also wrote about *expressive techniques* that are focused on body energy and movement in sessions. Given the lower potency of soft techniques, Smith viewed them as relatively safe compared to hard and expressive techniques, and I think this makes them preferable in psychoanalytic psychotherapy. In addition, softer techniques are often sufficient in trauma work without the need to move to harder or more expressive techniques. Many soft techniques overlap with containing–informing touch. For example, mutual hand holding or an embrace during an intense immersion in a trauma memory are types of touch that can provide both containment of the patient's emotions and also create an opportunity for the patient to discover and make use of their own agency.

Body psychotherapy is best learned through personal bodywork and study. Engaging in one's own bodywork with a trained body therapist deepens a therapist's understanding of their own body–mind connections. Such personal bodywork also reduces anxieties about touch with patients. For therapists who decide to make use of this form of touch with certain patients, I offer some suggestions in Chapter 4 about how to become more knowledgeable with these forms of touch.

Body Analysis

Body analysis is my preferred way of working physically with patients. This form of embodied therapy makes use of the other four categories of touch but includes a more intrapersonal and relational mix than the others. In this way, body analysis is a more comprehensive way of working with touch that begins after the patient and therapist have become comfortable working with the other categories of touch. In addition, body analysis occurs within three overlapping and non-linear phases. I categorize these phases as *regressive, transitional,* and *progressive.* In psychoanalysis, we speak of regressive and progressive phases of treatment. In self psychology, Tolpin (2002) speaks of both "trailing edge" and "forward edge" transferences (p. 168). In my work with embodied theory, I find a similarity between all three ways of tracking patient progress. I introduce my three phases here and discuss them throughout the book and in relation to cases.

Regressive Phase

The regressive phase speaks to work within embodied sensations and flash-backs related to the patient's trauma. When the abuse was in childhood, the emphasis will be on traumatized self states from childhood. If the abuse occurred in adulthood, the work addresses these specific adult self-states. The primary focus of the work is on the actual trauma experiences. It includes helping the patient develop a deeper understanding of the ways their traumas continue to disrupt and limit their relationship with their body. In psycho-analytic psychotherapy, heavy emphasis is often placed on regressive material, including child self-states, because many treatment issues have their origins in past experiences.

Transitional Phase

Movement out of the regressive into a more progressive phase often occurs within a transitional phase. In the transitional phase, the patient's fears and confusion around touch begin to give way to curiosity and desire for embo-died transformation. Their desire to reclaim their stolen body becomes central. This creates a shift from work that addresses the patient's trauma memories and flashbacks to helping the individual work toward developing a new and expansive relationship with their own body and the bodies of others as well. The patient becomes more curious about body and touch in ways that can be verbalized and explored in sessions. In the transitional phase, the patient can compare emotions and body sensations from the past with new ones emerging in the work with their therapist and in their personal relationships as well. For example, holding the therapist's hand in session can feel both anxiety provoking and liberating. The anxiety falls primarily within the regressive phase, while the liberating feelings signal a movement toward the progressive phase.

In an earlier model, I labeled this phase the *transgressive phase* because of the anxiety the patient may have when allowing themselves to feel their own embodied agency, aliveness, and pleasure. Often a patient reverts back to their trauma history and becomes anxious that there is something wrong with these feelings. I used the term transgressive to denote the patient's experience while being clear that this would not be an actual ethical transgression. Rather, the patient may feel they are transgressing, given they have generally avoided or been suspicious of these forms of touch following their abuse. I wrote, "The transgressive space is where the client's desire for change becomes verbalized and explored" (Novak, 2018, p. 290). I still believe this, but I now use the term transitional rather than transgressive to describe this phase because the former term fully encompasses both the patient's anxiety as well as their developing trust, confidence, and aliveness relative to touch. The transitional phase will be different for each patient depending on their own unique issues relative to body and touch.

Progressive Phase

In the progressive phase, the primary emphasis of the work is on helping the patient expand their ability to experience agency, aliveness, and pleasure in their body. Progressive work addresses both intrapersonal and relational embodied experiences, which includes embodied connections with others that can now feel enjoyable rather than terrifying or activating of a past trauma.

Even within the progressive phase, however, there are moments that can feel regressive or transgressive, especially early on in the shift out of the transitional phase. However, such moments carry less emotional intensity, are less frequent, and can be compared and contrasted to the new progressive feel of the body. In this way, the past history will continue to have a decreasing influence over how the patient relates to their own and others' bodies.

Like psychoanalytic psychotherapy, body analysis is generally a longer form of treatment. Working through a regressive–transitional–progressive embodied therapy requires months if not years of work depending on the patient's needs. Some embodied issues require a number of years of talk therapy before the patient and therapist reach the level of trust and under-standing that permits moving the therapy into specific embodied issues related to the patient's traumas.

Body analysis involves a methodical approach that is, in many ways, parallel to psychoanalytic psychotherapy. However, I use my training in psychoanalysis and my experiences of body analysis in all of my embodied work with patients, including short-term and symptom-relief treatments. A patient does not have to engage in a long-term analysis to reap benefits from working within a psycho-analytic frame. Similarly, once a therapist has developed the ability to work with body analysis, these skills can be modified, as appropriate, and used in work with all patients relative to the body, with and without touch.

The cases presented in Chapters 7 through 10 are examples of body analy-sis. They provide a detailed view of this systematic process and how embodied analysis makes use of the various categories of touch as the work moves through the three phases of treatment.

I think as the professions of psychoanalysis and psychotherapy become more accepting and knowledgeable of this type of work, there will be more theory, more practitioners, and a wider acceptance of its benefits. However, many clinicians who read this book will never want to work within a full body analysis with patients. In addition, not all patients need body analysis. Often, in trauma therapy, categories of touch such as completion touch and containing–informing touch can be enough to provide the patient with needed experiences of touch that can be processed in treatment. This can be espe-cially true of single-episode traumas or specific events within chronic trauma.

References

Boadella, D. (1987). *Life streams: An introduction to biosynthesis*. Routledge

Eldredge, C., & Cole, G. (2007). Learning from work with individuals with a history of trauma: Some thoughts on integrating body-oriented techniques and relational psychoanalysis. In F. S. Anderson (Ed.), *Bodies in treatment: The unspoken dimen-sion* (pp. 79–102). The Analytic Press.

Fonagy, P., Target, M., Gergely, G., & Jurist, E. (2002). *Affect regulation, mentaliza-tion, and the development of the self*. Other Press.

Holder, A. (2000). To touch or not to touch: That is the question. *Psychoanalytic Inquiry*, 20, 44–64. doi:10.1080/07351692009348874.

Keleman, S. (1975). *Your body speaks its mind*. Simon & Schuster.

Kelley, C. R. (1978). *Orgonomy, bioenergetics and radix: The Reichian movement today*. The Radix Institute.

Klopstech, A. (2009). So which body is it? The concepts of the body in psychotherapy. *Bioenergetic Analysis. The Clinical Journal of the International Institute for Bioe-nergetic Analysis*, 19, 11–30.

Lowen, A. (1975). *Bioenergetics*. Viking Penguin.

Novak, E. T. (2018). A model of informed physical contact in psychotherapy. *Trans-actional Analysis Journal*, 48(1), 18–32. doi:10.1080/03621537.2018.1397962.

Panksepp, J. (1998). *Affective neuroscience: The foundations of human and animal emotions.* Oxford University Press.

Reich, W. (1949). *Character analysis.* Orgone Institute Press.

Smith, E. W. L. (1985). *The body in psychotherapy.* McFarland & Company.

Stern, D. B. (2010). *Partners in thought: Working with unformulated experience, dissociation, and enactment.* Routledge.

Tolpin, M. (2002). Doing psychoanalysis of normal development: Forward edge transferences. *Progress in Self Psychology,* 18, 167–190. doi:10.4324/9780203780459.

Chapter 3

My Experience of Embodied Therapy

This chapter describes my experiences in what became two contrasting therapies: a classical psychoanalysis without touch and a body therapy with touch. More attention is given to my 5-year body therapy and the ways my massage therapist and I were able to make use of informed touch to reduce and even extinguish my embodied trauma flashbacks from childhood. This body therapy began during my first psychoanalysis and continued into a second one. Combining bodywork and a form of talk therapy can be controversial, although they have been addressed favorably elsewhere (Anderson, 2007). In my experience, they can provide a way for the patient to incorporate physical work into psychoanalytic treatment without direct touch from their therapist.

My intent is not to privilege my embodied therapy over analytic work. Rather, because this book is about embodied therapy, I want to emphasize that part of my own therapy. In addition, by providing an overview of some of my own bodywork, the reader will see how knowing my own traumas and body has been a critical component in using embodied therapy in my professional work with patients.

My Introduction to Body Psychotherapy

My professional interest in touch as a part of the therapeutic process began early in my career as I attempted to understand my own personal traumas, almost all of which occurred before the age of 7. The early absence of close bonding relationships with my parents and severe asthma that resulted in many hospitalizations before age 3 were then followed by sexual abuse between ages 4 and 6.

Each trauma created its own unique issues for me relative to my relationship with my own body and physical engagement with others. Like many abused individuals, I was unable to understand the links between my childhood trauma and my anxiety and fears around human physical contact. Forms of physical contact that would be welcomed and enjoyed by most people, such as hugs from friends or family, were always uncomfortable for

DOI: 10.4324/9781003215745-4

me. In my adolescence, desire for even mild consensual sexual engagements with girls my age always left me feeling like I was lecherous and had done something wrong.

My quest to reclaim my stolen body and to explore uninhibited pleasure in all forms of physical contact began in psychotherapy. I began a long-term psychotherapy based primarily on transactional analysis. Initially, the work addressed my issues of early parental separation and near fatal-asthma (NFA). I began to understand how these traumas were a major contributor to what had been a lifetime of intense anxiety and depression. I also began to understand that a form of bodywork would also be needed for my treatment.

My introduction to body psychotherapy came in the form of weekend workshops led by my therapist and his spouse. Those workshops focused on bodywork based primarily in neo-Reichian theory. The bodywork fell mostly within the category of somatic mastery and modulation and included both hard and soft techniques. Both leaders' backgrounds provided participants opportunities to process the bodywork within the framework of neo-Reichian, gestalt, transactional analysis, and other theories such as object relations.

The weekends were structured in a way that provided each participant with opportunities to address their specific body issues. This included times during which a group member could lay on a mat with a group leader kneeling next to them working directly with the participant's body. Several group members would also kneel around to offer interactive support. During my own "mat work," I discovered the ways my early attachment ruptures and asthma traumas could be accessed through embodied trauma memories that surfaced during the bodywork.

The safety of the group and use of physical contact during mat work—such as a hand on my shoulder, someone massaging my head, or a hand on my chest—offered me a containing space in which to relive many of the body sensations of my childhood asthma attacks. I could also feel and process my childhood abandonment with the group leader and other supportive coparticipants. At the time, I was unaware of my childhood sexual abuse, which I had involuntarily dissociated from cognitive memory. It would take almost another decade before a cognitive memory of that abuse surfaced.

Psychoanalysis without Touch

My years of psychotherapy and bodywork were followed by additional trauma work when I entered into my first classical psychoanalysis that began when I was also considering analytic training. As part of my analysis, I was encouraged to lie on the couch, which used to be a standard practice in psychoanalysis. However, I had difficulty moving from chair to couch sessions. Given my abuse history and knowledge of my body, I suspected lying on the couch would create intense embodied flashbacks that without physical contact for grounding might become overwhelming.

This was viewed by my analyst as my resistance to the process, a standard interpretation at the time. Even I considered the possibility that I was resisting lying on the couch as a form of defense rather than trusting my own knowledge of my self, my traumas, and my body. This situation was an example of a therapeutic mistake relative to my body that was occurring in a nontouch psychoanalysis. My analyst did not understand that my embodied isolation and abandonment in childhood had been so severe that revisiting those self-state experiences on the couch without some form of physical connection would lead to intense and unbearable embodied flashbacks.

Following months of conversation and encouragement for me to lie on the couch, I finally submitted to my analyst's preferred way of working. Even knowing the probability of an embodied trauma memory surfacing was high, I was overwhelmed by the intensity of what occurred. The moment I laid on the hard and rather unwelcoming couch, I could feel anxiety slowly begin to infiltrate every part of my body. From my years of body therapy, I knew how to stay with the anxiety and how to continue to observe and process the somatic sensations.

In my prior bodywork, when these embodied flashbacks occurred, someone would engage with me through either contact comfort or containing–informing touch. However, in the analysis, the classical approach of heavy silence and my analyst sitting behind me did not help me feel the connection that I desperately needed in order to stay grounded. My anxiety continued to increase and began to include somatic sensations, mostly connected to my NFA, including rapid breathing, trembling, and involuntary muscle spasms. In my own work with patients, I have found that patients with histories of embodied trauma often have symptoms of muscle spasms or ticks, often severe, that are similar to what I experienced in that first analysis.

In my case, I knew they were the result of embodied trauma memories from early childhood. However, I was unable to self-soothe or regulate them. In fact, I had never been able to do that effectively unless I was engaged in physical connection with someone. In retrospect, I am convinced that, regardless of the therapist, therapy on a couch without touch would have created a similar outcome for me. This intense reenactment required a form of physical connection to keep me anchored in the here and now. In my case, I do not believe a therapist's attempts at metaphorically "holding me" through eye contact, an empathic expression, or concerned look would have been enough to shift that torturous experience into something more manageable.

The regressive trauma reenactment and body memories intensified until they reached a point that I could not tolerate. My body was rising and writhing on the couch. I could feel the muscles around my rib cage expanding and contracting in the ways a body moves during an asthma attack. I sat up and spent the balance of the session working through hyperventilation and trying to recover my equilibrium. I was never able to effectively work on the couch without those embodied trauma memories surfacing and eventually spent the remainder of my time in analysis sitting up. The work of treating my embodied traumas stalled because, although we could talk about my traumas, the embodied work that was essential for my transformation was unavailable in that treatment. I had to look elsewhere and chose to return to a modality I had experienced some success with early in treatment: massage therapy.

Massage Therapy as a Form of Embodied Therapy

Because many of my traumas had occurred in infancy and early childhood, I needed a treatment that focused heavily on my embodied memories rather than on verbal narratives. Lauren was an experienced, licensed, talented massage therapist whose touch created a strong implicit connection with me. She and I worked within traditional massage therapy theory and technique, a framework many readers are likely familiar with. The session begins with the patient lying face up on the massage table, undressed and draped with a sheet. During the session, the body area to be worked on is uncovered while the rest remains covered.

During my early massages from Lauren, we began to lay the groundwork for the intense embodied therapy to follow. For many months we discussed my trauma history and issues around touch. At that point, many massages occurred with few words, and eye contact was limited because I closed my eyes in order to move more deeply into my internal states. In such treatment, although verbal interactions might help the patient feel grounded and keep them from becoming flooded with emotions (Ogden et al., 2006), especially early on, sometimes a fuller immersion is necessary to recognize, reclaim, and transform the body.

Because I had already spent years working on my traumas, and because Lauren was a skilled massage therapist, we were able to move quickly into a deeper immersion into my embodied memories and flashbacks. Her informed touch helped to create a nonverbal connection that provided me with a safe space to feel and remember I was not alone as I moved deeper into trauma memories. In this regressive phase, Lauren's touch fell more within the categories of containing–informing and contact comfort, helping me to stay connected to her without interrupting my deep internal reflection with words or eye contact.

The following example of my work begins in a regressive phase and illustrates how containing–informing physical contact can help a patient regulate intense affective and somatic memories. Eventually this regressive work can lead to a progressive phase and a deeper experience of a transformed self. The work described here occurred in year 2 of my work with Lauren.

I generally began the sessions within a present-day self-state experience. Lauren's touch was, at first, in the forefront of my mind as I reacquainted myself with her contact, voice, scent, and the space we were creating. After several minutes, I could relax and move into my own personal reverie, and my associations expanded to include scenes and self-states from my past. Here the session would move into a more regressive space. I would imagine and feel the emotions of sitting in my second-grade class, numb and missing my mother badly. I would feel the internal loss and confusion from that time as I visualized two different parts of my second-grade self, the internally confused and wounded boy and the outwardly confident boy I was at that age.

This reverie within my second-grade self-state would last several minutes or more and was followed by a shift into another memory from second grade. I thought about slicing my knee on the playground playing football and having to get eight stitches. The memories zoomed in on me sitting in the school office with my second-grade teacher. She was sitting beside me, comforting me, and my mind lingered on those feelings of comfort. I remembered the contrast of my painful injury and her gentle words and smile. I recalled how infrequently I felt that sort of compassion, which is probably why it still stood out so vividly. I would stay with these feelings for a while, wondering if this were a time to inform Lauren of these memories. I briefly became aware of her hands on my shoulders, her slow and steady breathing, and both the comforting and containing influence that her touch and presence were having on me. Her strong presence and attention reassured me that I was not alone in what was happening. I chose not to speak and would shift again to another memory. I envisioned my panicked and screaming mother and my distant father on the day I broke my elbow later that second-grade summer. I thought about the contrast between my parent's reaction to my arm and my teacher's responses to my knee. The former was a more common occurrence in my childhood, and the absence of felt empathy from my parents saddened me.

I stayed with the memories of my elbow surgery and hospital stay. The feelings of isolation and limited compassion triggered other associations. As I laid on the table, my shoulder would begin to twitch, signaling another movement back in time, and I noticed the adjustment in Lauren's hands. To be more connected to what was occurring in my body, she would reposition her hands from the top of my shoulders to underneath my back, supporting my shoulder blades. This shift signaled, without words or visual connection, that she too has noticed my regression into an early trauma memory as she had seen my body memories many times. She knew this form of embodied connection was a better match for what was surfacing. Her embodied attentiveness and connection permitted me to remain silent and continue moving deeper into my own experience.

From my years of therapy working on my childhood abandonment and asthma issues, I was quite familiar with my body memories. The twitch seemed to connect with my seven hospital stays for asthma, all before age 3. Having been able to recover the records of those stays, I even had some of the official hospital notes in my mind. Within the containing space of Lauren's hands, I was able to be curious about words that seemed to surface, such as, "was restless," "fussy," "cried," "ate jello," "placed in croupette," "sore throat," "difficulty breathing," and "adrenaline shot." They all seemed to be in sync with the body sensations beginning to surface in me while I was on the massage table. This was the beginning of a massive shift in the session.

My body sensations and involuntary muscle movements continued to intensify as my body began to recall what it was like struggling to breathe during an asthma attack. My calm reverie on the table would turn into something like a body nightmare as I began experiencing, in high definition, body memories of gasping for air. The embodied replay included my body stiffening, my shoulder blades turning inward in an attempt to expand my chest, and the muscles around my rib cage contracting to push air out of my lungs.

These sensations were similar to the ones I had experienced on the analytic couch. However, on the massage table, my violent body sensations were met with no words, only touch and Lauren's empathic presence. If anyone spoke it was usually me, something such as, "I hate this." My words were met with a physical response. One hand on my right shoulder blade, the other below the left side of my rib cage, moving in time with the movements of my terrified body. When my body trembled and I begin to rise off the table as if gasping for air, Lauren supported my back with both hands. This experience could last anywhere from 5 to 15 minutes and ended with me exhausted and collapsed on the table. But I was always relieved that Lauren had been able to witness and stay with me in my embodied flashback.

The balance of the session would shift back into a traditional massage and felt like a blend of contact comfort and completion touch as we processed the session. Lauren and I would both describe our understanding of my body movements, and I would recount what felt most helpful from her and what forms of memories surfaced for me during specific points in the flashback. Links between my body on the table and my childhood traumas were explored and possible adjustments to the work in the next session conceptualized.

As is the case in most bodywork and in psychoanalytic psychotherapy, the processing was asymmetrical and focused on me as the patient. Lauren rarely disclosed what her own personal experience may have been, and I rarely asked. However, over the years of working together, I had come to know a good deal about her experience, implicitly through her empathic and attuned physical connection with me.

The session just described was not a one-time, corrective experience. These body sessions, like any work with trauma, occurred over months. During this regressive phase, for over 6 months, we met twice a week. My early traumas became known to me in ways I could never have imagined or probably ever wanted to know, even though I needed to. Each session presented a new body nuance for me to pay attention to and created links to how they were still being played out in my current life. The physical engagement with Lauren provided me with both explicit and implicit connections with a trusted other. This helped me stay within the feelings and sensations of past traumas without fearing I would become stuck, overwhelmed, and alone within the trauma replays.

Following months of this work, I was ready and wanted to reduce or even extinguish those embodied memories and reactions. This signaled a shift into a more progressive phase that began to help me reconfigure and transform my embodied trauma memories. I requested that if Lauren was willing, rather than supporting my back when I began to lift off the table, she would instead gently hold my shoulders down. I thought her hands would provide a form of reassurance that everything was OK, she was with me, and there was no reason for me to rise up on the table because I was not in danger of being unable to breathe. I thought that this nonverbal reassurance would help slow down my ingrained embodied reaction, keep my back on the table, and eventually reduce those embodied memories. And that is exactly what happened. This work could be categorized as somatic mastery and modulation, a rare time in our work when we shifted from soft techniques and used a mild form of the hard techniques defined in Chapter 2.

After further discussions about how to proceed, Lauren cautiously agreed and was willing to provide firm but not hard pressure (which she felt could have been misinterpreted as abusive by my child self-state). Her hands on my shoulders and the firm pressure were enough to encourage me and my body to trust that I could stay flat on the table when those memories surfaced. Again, no words were necessary until afterward when we processed the experience. One adjustment we made to the exercise was that I placed my hands on top of hers. This was a form of containing touch that helped me feel more connected to her. In addition, this increased my sense of adult agency. Rather than actually being a helpless infant, I was an adult man actively contributing to transforming my embodied trauma. With repeated sessions, my embodied trauma memories and triggers relative to my childhood asthma attacks were extinguished. I no longer feel panic when faced with situations I used to fear for lack of oxygen (e.g., swimming underwater, unventilated rooms, running, turtlenecks, head colds, etc.). This work also ended years of body unrest that I had erroneously diagnosed as generalized anxiety. I now understood how a major part of my intense anxiety had been linked to my infancy all along.

Applications to Psychoanalytic Psychotherapy

My own experience working with a massage therapist is something most therapists will not be able to provide for their patients. However, therapists can still make use of this example, as I do, when working within a psychoanalytic psychotherapeutic setting. In my own embodied treatment, the primary touch was containing–informing. My massage therapist followed my body's lead and responded to it. Touch was shoulder blades, rib cage, shoulders, and hand on chest. These are body areas I have also worked with in sessions with patients needing embodied trauma therapy.

Lauren's touch was not intended to primarily provide symptom relief or gratify a childhood need, although both of those did occur in the work. Primarily, however, Lauren's physical connections were in the service of the transformation of my embodied trauma memories.

In addition, the work was not designed to, nor did it, shift me into a sexualized experience of Lauren. Given the understandable professional and societal fears of touch in treatment, the pleasure I experienced in having an attractive woman's warm, soft hand firmly holding my hand or touching me as I lay on the massage table could raise some suspicions. However, within the context of these sessions, that was the only thing I found pleasurable about moving back into embodied flashbacks of childhood terrors. Lauren's informed physical connections allowed me to tolerate a deeper immersion into those embodied flashbacks. The work was also primarily focused on my own body rather than on the relational mix between our bodies.

In psychoanalytic psychotherapy, sitting shoulder to shoulder or holding hands could be enough to create this form of safe, sacred space and connection for the patient. Their experience might be described as a form of internal free association in the context of which the patient can explore multiple somatic sensations and specific self-states while anchored to their therapist through the physical connection. The therapist can also notice the patient's specific somatic sensations (e.g., shallow breathing, a leg twitch, hands clenching, etc.). Over time, the therapist learns how somatic movements are connected to the patient's specific self-states and how best to relate to the person in such moments.

The sustained embodied engagement with the therapist can also act as a continued nonverbal reminder that the patient is in a safe space with their trusted therapist. The patient experiences a "the coast is clear" situation in which a trauma memory is not going to pop up and hijack them. In this space, they can relax within their own body

In my own work, a more progressive and relational treatment began when the therapy shifted from working on my infant traumas to addressing my early childhood sexual abuse. The sexual abuse memories surfaced only after the work on my infant traumas was almost complete. In the section that follows, I briefly review relational embodied theory before moving into a clinical example based on my own sexual abuse therapy.

The Relational Embodied Experience

Klopstech (2009) has noted that the more relational theories of psychoanalysis have expanded to focus more on the two bodies in the consulting room along with the two subjectivities. She wrote about what she referred to as "the relational body in psychoanalysis" (p. 20), where not only the two minds but the two bodies are intersubjectively entwined, and referenced analysts such as Aron (1998), Harris (1998), and Dimen (1998) who all wrote about this relational body. However, these writings are generally still focused on nontouch treatments.

On the other hand, some therapists have written about their own relational experiences with touch. In the self psychology community, even Kohut's (2010) two fingers of touch produced results that were unexpected, unimagined (and probably not fully understood) within his working relationship with a patient. Other therapists have written about significant moments with touch in treatment, including in their own analysis (Bacal, 2011) or with patients (Cornell, 2015; McLaughlin, 2000; Mintz, 1969).

In my own bodywork, at the relational level, physical connections resonated differently for various self-states. Over the 5 years of embodied treatment with Lauren, her touch evoked many different reactions in me. From within a regressed frame, these were more within the terrain of projection and transference. In regressive moments, I could experience her and her touch as mothering, perhaps the cool babysitter I never had during my preadolescent years, a first infatuation, even a first high school sweetheart. Exploring my projections and transference in similar ways to psychoanalytic processing provided me with insights into how my early traumas had influenced the ways I related to many different people in my life. Over time, my experience of Lauren became more anchored in the present, progressive embodied experience we were creating.

The shift into a more progressive phase was preceded by a transitional phase as our embodied interactions brought right into the massage session the relational terror of touch I often felt when in physical contact with a woman. My issues with physical contact were deeply ingrained and organized within procedural memory that had never been amendable to transformation in any form of nontouch treatment.

My bodywork occurred at the same time my analysis was sinking deeper into a lengthy and traumatic impasse. The absence of touch, along with a strict adherence to classic psychoanalytic theory and methodology, contributed to intense reenactments. My requests for touch were met with anxious rejection and classical interpretations that seemed to blame me rather than accurately address what was going on. This only confirmed my worst fear: that there was something evil or lecherous about me, otherwise my analyst would not be so terrified of touching me. I moved into a deep regressive phase that I could not pull myself out of or find relief from.

Mintz (1969) postulated that her own touch of a patient acted as a "symbol of acceptance" (p. 373) that reduced her patient's overwhelming sense of shame and embarrassment, a situation that could have ended treatment. The symbol of acceptance was necessary to combat the patient's sense of being physically repulsive. Mintz was also convinced that in this specific case "verbal communication in itself could not have alleviated the agonizing sense of worthlessness" (p. 374).

In my own analysis, any of the categories of touch would have helped, including something as simple as a pass-by handshake, to provide me with concrete evidence that my analyst was not afraid of me as some form of perverse man. In retrospect, I was actually experiencing myself within my 6-year-old belief that I was a child who sexually abuses women merely with his touch. The "no touch" therapeutic frame confirmed my belief that my touch was perverse and damaging and intensified my heightened fears and shame that I was a lecherous person.

These issues also began to seep into my work and relationship with Lauren. Perhaps our most important relational work with touch occurred during the transitional phase, during which there were times when I had difficultly believing touch between us was permissible and consensual. My enjoyment and pleasure of her innocent therapeutic touch had me suspicious of my possible "unconscious" motivations, which I feared were more lecherous than my overt therapeutic motivations. On a few occasions, I even felt her touch as suspicious. In this transitional phase, I simultaneously experienced our embodied connections as progressively therapeutic while at the same time feeling regressive apprehension that this touch would be interpreted as abusive, with me being blamed and seen as a pervert.

A vignette from my work in this transitional space illustrates how we were able to work through my relational confusions about touch. It highlights the transformations that occurred for me at both explicit and implicit levels of organization and the changes that occurred in my ingrained patterns of relating to another's touch. The work started in a more regressive phase, moved through a transitional phase, and ended within a more progressive phase.

This work took place several years into treatment and followed the bodywork discussed earlier in this chapter. That work had focused on my traumas before age 3. The newfound clarity about my early life seemed to allow memories of sexual abuse between the ages of 4 and 6 to begin to surface. In that abuse I had been set up as the perpetrator (i.e., the one touching and "wanting" to touch). Also, my abuser was female, and sadly my mother, who was unconsciously reenacting her own childhood abuse. In my work with Lauren I began understanding how for years somatic sensations and anxiety around touch that I had attributed to my NFA were actually related to my sexual abuse.

The previously dissociated or split-off experiences of childhood sexual abuse were now available in fragmented cognitive memories and intense body sensations. I suddenly had more difficulty with just about all forms of touch, and my past anxieties around even social touch began to make more sense. I also became an absolute believer in both the existence of repressed memory and Schwartz's (2000) conviction that the most common form of false memory is "fabricated memories of nonabuse" (p. 26).

One day I arrived for a session with Lauren immediately following a disruptive analytic session. I was still somewhat disorganized in my thinking, and I was hoping there would be a way for Lauren to help me get myself back together. However, in the state I was in, I did not trust even her. In that moment, she was a suspicious stand-in for my mother. I asked Lauren if we could just sit on the massage table next to one another and hold hands. I was not sure at the time why I was unwilling to lie on the table or why I was making my request. Generally, having no idea why a patient wants a certain type of touch, especially when they are in some form of dissociated or traumatized self-state, is not informed touch, and my massage therapist empathically attempted to understand why I wanted that form of connection. Unfortunately, I could not explain my motivations because I was too panicked, ashamed, and confused. She appropriately and gently rejected my request and wanted to talk more about what was going on for me, given both my and now her confusion over what was happening.

Her informed "no touch" response was not easy for me to take. Despite her best efforts to reassure me that she was not offended or frightened by my request, I now felt more panic, suspicion, and shame. Both my analyst and now my massage therapist seemed to confirm that my simple requests for touch were actually some form of perversive act. I believed that I was being seen as, or was becoming, the feared perpetrator I had been made out to be in childhood. I canceled my appointments with Lauren for over a month, assuring her that she had done nothing wrong. I returned only after a cool-down period. I also ended my analysis and began analysis with a psychoanalyst more familiar with embodied trauma.

A month later, back in session with Lauren, we were able to process, repair, and then later reconfigure this part of myself and our relationship. We discovered that we were apparently in the eye of my sexual abuse storm, and we spent the next several months navigating through that regressive phase together. I would also take our work back to my new analyst for continued processing.

This period was the only time when Lauren's touch was confusing to me in ways that made me question whether it was appropriate for us to continue with our work. I even thought that maybe I needed a male massage therapist, given my issues of sexual abuse by a female. Fortunately, the trust Lauren and I had developed within our working relationship helped us to continue the work.

A breakthrough came one day as I lay on the table; I recovered explicit details of my sexual abuse, which I had never before recalled. During a period of internal reverie mixed with terror, while Lauren held my head in her hands, I recalled, in high definition, the before, during, and after of one of my childhood sexual abuse scenes. This is not an uncommon occurrence within embodied treatment, and containing–informing touch can often help the patient feel connected to their therapist within the intensity of the memory. In my case, as Lauren held my head, I noticed two things that were different about the memories now available to me.

First, previously remembered fragments of the incident were connecting with these new parts of memory, and they were triggering other fragments of new memories. These new details helped create this complete sexual abuse scene.

Second, and strangely, as I replayed the memory in my mind, watching myself being abused, I noticed that standing in the bedroom with me was a second person, a witness: Lauren. In my fantasy she was witnessing the abuse. This made sense at the time in that we had been working on my abuse for years and had worked through fragmented abuse scenes. My body was now telling an abuse scene without any words, and Lauren was implicitly in tune with my body's nonverbal narrative. The ability of the patient to tell a trauma experience only through their body, and the therapist's ability to observe and respond with embodied empathy, is a significant transformative event in embodied trauma work. As the memory continued, I began to feel intensifying shame, fear, and disgust, which all crescendoed to a point that was intolerable for me. Lauren's touch went from comforting to confusing and feeling almost incestuous, and I requested that she stop all contact.

That was a significant moment in our work. Even then I remember reflecting on how at one level I was aware that she was my well-trusted and trained massage therapist and that what was going on for me was an embodied flashback. Yet, even the awareness of our therapeutic relationship was not enough to counter the strong reactions coming from within my somatic memories of childhood abuse. This is one reason why in embodied work it is essential that the patient can stop touch at any time and that the therapist comply with such a request.

This experience has served me well with many of my own patients. Specifically, when our embodied connection contributes to the patient becoming flooded in a flashback, I am more aware of when to continue the embodied connection and when to physically disengage. In addition, if the patient abruptly moves away from me, frightened of me and my touch, I can remain a present and calming figure who can help them process and move out of the heightened anxiety, even though we are no longer physically connected.

For example, at one point Lauren removed her hands from underneath my head and moved a chair several feet from the table. I could see the look of empathic concern—not panic, anger, or repulsion—in her eyes. I recounted to her in detail what I had just remembered. Her moist eyes metaphorically embraced me as we felt this past trauma together. The session ended with me extending my hand and her moving to take it (completion touch) as we both honored in silence for several minutes what we had uncovered and experienced together.

Our trauma work at an embodied relational level allowed for reconfiguring my own understandings of my childhood traumas and my relationships to physical engagement with others. This helped me not only to be less anxious about physical contact with other people but also to be able to even find pleasure in touch. When I was not in her office, I began to notice that within my memories of trauma, my witness, Lauren, had been integrated into those memories. Remarkably, my trauma history now had not only a partner in thought (Stern, 2010) but a partner in emotions and body. The full immersion into my past traumas had "photoshopped" Lauren into the memories. To this day, my trauma memories do not propel me back into the past. Rather, they are housed within Lauren's office. Gone are hospital cribs and adult bedrooms. These have been replaced by a healing massage table and a loving massage therapist: a tragically beautiful experience.

References

Anderson, F. S. (2007). *Bodies in treatment: The unspoken dimension*. The Analytic Press.

Aron, L. (1998). The clinical body and the reflexive mind. In F. S. Anderson & L. Aron (Eds.), *Relational perspectives on the body* (pp. 3–38). The Analytic Press.

Bacal, H. A. (2011). *The power of specificity in psychotherapy: When therapy works and when it doesn't*. Jason Aronson.

Cornell, W. F. (2015). *Somatic experience in psychoanalysis and psychotherapy: In the expressive language of the living*. Routledge.

Dimen, M. (1998). Polyglot bodies: Thinking through the relational. In F. S. Anderson & L. Aron (Eds.), *Relational perspectives on the body* (pp. 65–93). The Analytic Press.

Harris, A. (1998). Psychic envelopes and sonorous baths: Siting [sic] the body in relational theory and clinical practice. In F. S. Anderson & L. Aron (Eds.), *Relational perspectives on the body* (pp. 39–64). The Analytic Press.

Klopstech, A. (2009). So which body is it? The concepts of the body in psychotherapy. *Bioenergetic Analysis: The Clinical Journal of the International Institute for Bioenergetic Analysis*, 19, 11–30.

Kohut, H. (2010). On empathy: Heinz Kohut (1981). *International Journal of Psychoanalytic Self Psychology*, 5(2), 122–131. doi:10.1080/15551021003610026.

McLaughlin, J. T. (2000). The problem and place of physical contact in analytic work: Some reflections on handholding in the analytic situation. *Psychoanalytic Inquiry*, 20(1), 65–81. doi:10.1080/07351692009348875.

Mintz, E. E. (1969). Touch and the psychoanalytic tradition. *Psychoanalytic Review*, 56(3), 365–376. doi:10.1037/h0088759.

Ogden, P., Minton, K., & Pain, C. (2006). *Trauma and the body: A sensorimotor approach to psychotherapy*. W.W. Norton.

Schwartz, H. L. (2000). *Dialogues with forgotten voices: Relational perspectives of child abuse trauma and treatment of dissociative disorders*. Basic Books.

Stern, D. B. (2010). *Partners in thought: Working with unformulated experience, dissociation, and enactment*. Routledge.

Chapter 4

Training, Study, and the Art of Embodied Therapy

Whenever I present to groups or speak with colleagues about my model of embodied therapy, there is always deep respect for the therapeutic benefits of such work. But when I suggest it can become an integral part of psychoanalytic psychotherapy with trauma patients, there is an almost predictable hesitation and caution and the strong sense that embodied therapy requires special training before a therapist should engage in it with patients.

Nevertheless, as already discussed, many therapists do engage in some forms of physical contact with some patients such as pass-by handshakes and completion touch hugs or even forms of containing–informing touch, despite having no exposure to training or study in embodied therapy. Perhaps because handshakes and hugs are familiar social forms of physical engagement, these feel safer. But safe and familiar does not equate to therapeutically effective or knowing how to then process the interaction. Even these social forms of physical engagement need to be understood within a model of embodied therapy.

This chapter suggests some elements that might be included in independent study relative to integrating touch into treatment. Each therapist needs to decide for themselves what types of touch they want to incorporate into treatment and the appropriate level of study required for it. In addition, different licensure boards and professional organizations may have their own rules and criteria for the use of touch, and therapists should familiarize themselves with those as part of their studies.

The depth of study also needs to be based on how a therapist wants to make use of touch in their practice. For some therapists, work with touch will be focused more on symptom relief and how to manage trauma or embodied flashbacks. This would mean working primarily with completion touch and containing–informing touch. Other therapists may want to work with patients beyond symptom relief in attempts to transform the person's embodied trauma and traumatized self-states. Embodied therapy in these instances would then fall further on the continuum into somatic mastery and modulation and body analysis. For this type of work, a therapist should acquire more extensive understanding of trauma theory and embodied work.

DOI: 10.4324/9781003215745-5

Currently, the study of embodied therapy requires stepping outside of the psychotherapeutic or psychoanalytic communities. A good starting point for therapists interested in exploring professional training is the United States Association for Body Psychotherapy (USABP). My own training has been a never-ending and expansive independent study. The primary components have been seminars on touch and body processes, individual and group consultations with an emphasis on bodywork, a year in massage school that did not lead to licensure but provided me with some basics relative to body and touch, and, of course, my own bodywork, primarily on massage tables and in weekend workshops.

The Therapist's Own Body and Personal Embodied Work

Personal bodywork expands a clinician's relationship with their own body and helps them understand their own strengths, limits, and therapeutic style of working with embodied issues both with and without touch. It also provides an opportunity for them to analyze how their own histories of touch with caregivers influences the ways they engage in or avoid certain types of touch and how this may play out in embodied work with patients.

The study of bodywork is similar to psychoanalytic psychotherapy training in that one of the most important components of analytic training is the candidate's own training analysis. Similarly, engaging in forms of personal bodywork is the bedrock of a therapist's training in embodied therapy.

Embodied interactions with trained professionals expand the therapist's understanding of both sides of the embodied relationship. Clinical issues that are common to psychoanalytic psychotherapy are also part of embodied work. These included transference and countertransference, projection, enactments, reenactments, rupture, and repair. In personal embodied work, these issues are experienced first hand, thus providing insights and perspectives that help therapists develop their own embodied treatment style.

In personal embodied work, a therapist experiences how initiating and receiving touch evokes multiple reactions from within their different self-states at different times. This helps them gain an understanding of when certain types of physical engagement might be motivated more by their own needs rather than the patient's and what might prevent or motivate them to include touch with a specific patient.

Personal embodied work can be done with professionals such as body therapists, massage therapists, and clinicians who have experience in embodied therapy. In addition to individual work, the ability to work within a group can be quite informative. I also know clinicians who have included yoga and dance—such as Argentine tango, which is improvisational and intimate—in their personal embodied work to enhance their relationship and understanding of their body.

Therapists should expect to work with several different body therapists in their training. For example, working with body therapists within and across one's gender identity expands a therapist's understanding of how the dynamics of touch can change depending on the genders of both the patient and the therapist. Finding one person who can work across various nuanced forms of physical connection can be difficult, especially in terms of the more relational forms of work with embodied trauma.

In my personal work, there was considerable trial and error involved in finding massage therapists who were a good fit for the work I needed at certain times. One evening at dinner, a good friend was suffering the normal back tightness of middle age and asked if I knew a good massage therapist. Before I could respond, my wife joked, "Of course he does. Ed has had a massage from about every massage therapist in Ohio!" Sometimes this felt true. I needed to work with body specialists who could help me understand the impact initiating and receiving touch would have on my infant, child, and adult self-states, both traumatized and nontraumatized ones. Often, the person I found for this work was someone who had been physically or sexually abused themselves and also wanted to learn more about their own embodied issues. In these instances, we were able to engage in more mutual embodied explorations that were generally still asymmetrically tilted toward my issues. Although I was the client, we could still explore and process the mutual impact of our embodied work.

Following my own independent study, I found that, for the first time in my life, I could be fully engaged and present for meaningful embraces with family, friends, and even my wife and son. Most noticeable was how I could hug nephews and nieces without apprehension. Sadly, by the time I had completed this work, many years and many opportunities for hugs had been lost. These losses remain a personal reminder of the importance of this work.

As the clinician becomes more knowledgeable and comfortable with embodied therapy, practicing with another colleague may be possible and can enhance both clinicians' confidence and comfort with touch. Two colleagues taking turns at being the therapist and patient in a form of embodied role play, and their processing of these exercises, deepens their understanding of embodied therapy. For example, the two colleagues could sit on the couch holding hands and explore and process what this feels like and evokes in them and what might occur with specific patients.

Making Therapeutic Use of Personal Bodywork

Personal bodywork helps the clinician develop clarity around their own embodied boundaries in ways that make it easier to then devote full embodied attentiveness to the patient without fear of overstepping or moving into a possible boundary violation. The clinician's calmness, confidence, and reverence for embodied therapy is essential for the patient to be able to trust and to also feel trusted by the therapist.

The therapist will also be able to notice and understand what is going on much more quickly and to anticipate what is and is not optimal for the patient. When mistakes or misattunements occur, the therapist is more likely to pick up on them quickly and understand what adjustments are necessary without becoming flooded with their own fears or anxiety. This is not possible if the therapist has not experienced their own embodied work as part of their training.

Personal embodied work also helps the therapist become comfortable with the mutual embodied influence patient and therapist have on one another. In embodied therapy, especially body analysis, the patient is both receiving and initiating forms of physical engagement and will learn a good deal about both their own body and the therapist's. Working body to body makes it more difficult for the therapist to conceal their own embodied reactions, which are an important part of embodied therapy. Trauma patients can sense they are having an impact on the therapist that does not lead to the patient being abused, exploited, or blamed for some type of boundary violation. This reduces the patient's fears and confusions around touch. The therapist generally does not go into much detail about their embodied experience, but when processing they can confirm or adjust the patient's assessment of how the therapist was experiencing the session relative to both the patient's and their own body.

I believe a reason embodied therapy can be anxiety provoking for the therapist is that the patient is going to come to know the therapist's body to some extent. In this way they improve their capacity to trust their own perceptions of physical engagements, without reflexively moving into a default position of fear and suspicion. The patient's ability to trust their own perceptions of physical contact is a central component in the transformative properties of embodied therapy.

My patients notice what is going on in my body when we are physically engaged. They can also intuitively pick up on when I may be unclear about what I think might be the best form of physical connection at a given time, especially when we are in the initial stages of embodied work. This usually registers as my being careful and respecting the sacredness of the work. Early in embodied therapy, patients are also more focused on how my touch is not sexual or exploitive and that my body is not aroused by the work. Many are often amazed at how their own experience is not sexual. This can be a truly remarkable moment for patients who were sexually abused in childhood and have lived with the belief and fear that all touch will turn sexual.

As the work in embodied therapy progresses, the patient may notice moments of erotic aliveness that fall on a continuum. The pleasure of physical engagement, without acting out, is a turning point for many patients. This progressive work allows the patient, often for the first time since their abuse, to create a continuum of pleasurable touch without fearing or believing all pleasure in touch will be sexualized. The meaning of physical touch radically changes and expands, with the patient contrasting their embodied memories of abuse with the embodied sense of safety, relaxation, and pleasure in the therapeutic moment.

Supervision and Consultation

Working with patients in embodied therapy requires the clinician to, at times, make use of other therapists' minds and bodies to help them process the treatment. Bollas (2013) wrote how in psychoanalytic psychotherapy consultation with other colleagues can also provide a supportive "holding environment" (p. 53) for the therapist. This is also true for embodied work. Personally, there is no way I would work with physical contact beyond completion touch without some form of consultation. However, I would also not work in traditional psychoanalysis without consultation.

For most therapists, becoming comfortable presenting their embodied work in traditional supervision, consultation, or a study group can take some time and may feel quite vulnerable. I am always reminded of my own early anxiety when younger therapists express their fears and concerns in presenting their work to me. The anxiety can intensify when the case includes some form of misattunement, mistake, or enactment.

Consultations about embodied work involving physical contact can create even more intense anxiety. The professional stigma around touch can lead to suspicion around the use of therapeutic touch, let alone touch that creates a form of enactment, reenactment, or rupture. In addition, to effectively process an embodied experience, the consultee needs to provide detailed information about the physical interactions that occurred. Most therapists are not used to presenting or consulting in such detail, and it requires some getting used to for both the therapist and the consultant or study group. This is because it is not enough to talk about the actual touch between patient and therapist. There are many more details, such as issues of transference and countertransference, that need to be addressed as well as areas of exploration and processing such as smells and scent. A patient and therapist sitting in physical proximity makes different types of smells accessible: sometimes the pleasant smell of a patient's minty toothpaste, other times the garlic from their lunch. Conversely, the patient is picking up various scents from the analyst as well—in my case, probably the smell of the many coffees I have had during the day.

Another issue is that because there are so few therapists who actually work with physical interactions, finding an appropriate, useful consultant can be difficult. Again, moving outside of psychoanalysis or psychotherapy to consult with body psychotherapists or even massage therapists, as appropriate, may be useful.

Body-to-body consultations allow the therapist to explore the kinds of touch that are occurring with a patient so that the therapist develops a clearer understanding of what that touch might feel like to the person. For example, I have sometimes consulted with massage therapists who touch me in a certain way a patient likes to be touched. Thus I learn in a direct way what the patient may be experiencing.

I was fortunate to have both individual and group consultations that combined psychoanalytic psychotherapy and embodied therapy with specific patients. Several of the members of our study group were also engaged in forms of physical work with some patients, and attention to body process with and without touch was a central part of our study. We also presented cases in which engaging in bodywork with a patient was being contemplated. More times than not, the group recommended against moving into touch with the patient, often because it was too soon in the treatment rather than not appropriate. However, even when the sense of the group was to avoid or delay touch, the therapist benefitted from presenting and exploring their motivations for wanting to include embodied therapy and thinking about the patient's embodied issues within the group process. The individual and group consultations helped me to feel more confident in moving from the basics of embodied therapy into deeper ways of working with embodied processes and were important in my development of the model described in this book.

I was also fortunate to have as a supervisor in my psychoanalytic training and then later as a consultant an analyst who could process my embodied work with patients. Despite no formal training in embodied therapy, her studies, teaching, and writing on many topics and theories were a natural match for processing my embodied work with patients. These include mother/infant research, attachment theory, and empathic attunement in relation to the theory of self psychology. With her, I presented cases that included embodied therapy, and we processed them within the context of many theories.

A final note on consultation: I always advise patients in embodied therapy that I will be consulting our work. I want the patient, or their child self-states, to hear that our work with touch will not be a secret. This is to deliberately contrast it with most childhood abuse, in which victims are told not to tell anyone and threatened with serious consequences to themselves and others if they do. In addition, I often take parts of the consultation back to the patient to continue processing with them. Patients appreciate that the work is being treated with this level of seriousness and reverence.

The Art of Using Touch

In psychoanalytic training we learn about many theories and constructs, such as confrontation, interpretation, enactments, transference and countertransference, dream interpretation, neuroscience, and so on. The therapist then has to develop their own ability to know when and how to make use of their training with specific patients. That is why psychoanalysis is sometimes referred to as an art. But just as having a palette loaded with paint does not make someone an artist, having a "palette" of embodied techniques does not make someone good at embodied therapy. The therapist needs to develop an understanding of what a patient needs and when they need it. In this way, embodied therapy can make use of Bacal's (2011) thinking that "therapeutic possibility is co-created in the specificity of fit between the patient's particular therapeutic needs and that therapist's capacity to respond to them, both of which will emerge and change within the unique process of each particular dyad" (p. 267). This specificity is part of the art of touch, especially in body analysis.

The Anticipation of Touch

When working with physical contact, the patient should always be able to anticipate the therapist's touch. This is another reason why massage is such a good way to introduce a traumatized body to safe touch. In a standard massage, the client can anticipate where the massage therapist's hands will move next. Generally, a massage starts with the client facing upward. The massage progresses head to shoulders, arms, hands, legs, and feet. The standard process provides consistency that keeps the patient from being surprised or startled by touch because they generally know which part of their body will be touched next.

Similar to massage, embodied work in psychoanalytic psychotherapy uses a personalized form of predictable touch based on the patient's needs. Each session generally begins the same way (e.g., sitting on chairs holding hands, sitting side by side on the couch, or sitting apart prior to engaging in touch). At the beginning of the session, the patient will inform the therapist of anything they are feeling that needs to be addressed or avoided in the session. In this way the patient helps to structure the work, thereby increasing the likelihood that they and their therapist will be able to anticipate how touch will occur. In the initial stages of therapy, even before touch is incorporated into treatment, the patient and therapist will explore what they are anticipating touch will evoke. Over time there is generally less need for detailed processing before a session, although the level of processing during the embodied experience will fluctuate. However, there is almost always processing afterward or at the beginning of the next session.

In my own work with patients, touch during the regressive phase is always more planned out and predictable. In the transitional phase, there are usually moments of spontaneous touch that blend in with the more structured physical contact. However, even these spontaneous moments can be implicitly anticipated by both patient and therapist. A patient's ability to move into initiating and receiving spontaneous touch can be an indication that the person is moving into a more progressive phase. As would be expected, in the progressive phase the touch becomes even more spontaneous because the patient and therapist have over many months, if not years, created a predictable and consistent routine around the use of touch. They have worked together long enough that each can anticipate what is going to occur based on the history of the work. I have compared this more spontaneous work to the trust and skill of a high-wire act team: two circus trapeze performers high above the ground, both having total trust that the other knows the routine, and each can anticipate the other's ways of moving. This too is the art in embodied therapy.

Hugs

I end this chapter addressing patient and therapist hugs, the form of physical connection I hear about most in consultation, even from therapists who say they do not work with embodied therapy. The consultations are either about a hug that has already occurred or one a patient has been requesting, with the therapist considering whether to accommodate the request.

In such consultations, the therapist is often seeking some form of permission or reassurance that I believe a hug was or will be therapeutic. Rather than focusing primarily on the "hug or not hug" question, consultations need to explore issues such as the possible motivations for the hug, how to structure it, and what the therapist is anticipating the hug will feel like and evoke in the patient and in themselves.

An issue generally not well thought out prior to consultation is whether the hug is expected to be a one-time physical interaction or one of several or many. In my own work, if a patient requests one hug and no more, I am always curious as to why they are requesting it. I generally ask questions such as what is motivating the request, what are they are hoping to experience from the hug, what do they not want to experience, would they prefer a firm or soft embrace, and so on. After we have processed, if we are both comfortable we usually engage in the hug. Sometimes, but not often, after processing the patient changes their mind and decides either to wait until more therapy has taken place or not to hug at all.

In the case of a request for a more spontaneous completion hug at the end of a session, especially after intense work, the therapist will need to make use of their own understanding of the therapeutic benefits and possible risks of the hug, as well as the patient's and their own motivations, to inform them about whether or not to hug. When I do deny a request for a hug, I generally offer a handshake and an explanation then, or in the next session, for my decision.

What I almost never do is initiate a hug with a patient. In my first 5 years as a therapist, I would occasionally offer a hug to someone whom I sensed might want to engage in a completion touch hug after an intense session. I was unaware of the bind this creates for the patient. With my offer, the hug became mine, not theirs. The patient was usually conflicted because a part of them wanted the hug while another part did not. I naïvely privileged the part that wanted the hug while dismissing the more cautious part. I was also unaware of how some patients could be worried about disappointing me if they rejected my offer. In addition, I was dismissing the need to process even supposedly simple things like an innocent and empathic hug.

These issues became clearer in a consultation I received about a female patient to whom I had offered such a hug. She apprehensively declined. In consultation, we processed issues such as those just described, and I was educated on how complicated a decision this would have been for that patient based on her issues. From that day forward, I have been less inclined to offer spontaneous hugs.

Another issue I had been blind to was that just because I was the therapist, I was not in some special category that meant I would be trusted. I did not yet understand how I could be viewed as suspicious with possible ulterior motives, especially by the patient's traumatized self-states. After all, many patients were abused by a parent, relative, or trusted family friend. The fact I was a licensed therapist was not an automatic reason to trust me with touch.

When hugs become part of treatment, they can also move beyond completion touch into containing–informing (with an emphasis on informing) and even somatic mastery and modulation and body analysis. The patient and therapist can also explore the possibility of the hug occurring during the session so that time can be spent processing rather than always at the end when time does not permit detailed processing.

In this type of work with hugs, the patient can become more curious and notice things at embodied levels that are then processed; for example, when and how they become more comfortable with hugs or if they remain somewhat anxious about them. Either the patient or the therapist might decide that the work with hugs is not creating the therapeutic benefits that had been anticipated, and then they can decide whether to continue them or not.

Over time, a hug may feel more like an embrace as the patient holds it longer. Sometimes it may be softer, other times firmer. Such variations can be processed in terms of how the patient experiences them. A chin may rest on a shoulder, a cheek may touch a cheek, the patient may smell the therapist's shampoo, perfume, deodorant, or breath. Being curious about such subtle nuances can lead to links and associations that provide the patient with more insight and experience relative to their body in both regressive and progressive states of being.

The work with hugs can often lead into even more expansive uses of embodied therapy, such as sitting next to one another in chairs, and can be a way of slowly expanding embodied work. Sitting next to each other in chairs is often how I begin embodied treatment. I have two large leather chairs that I move side by side so that there is still body separation but arms and hands can rest on the arm rests. From there the patient can initiate connections of hands and arms within the safe and firm boundary of the chairs. In such a heavily boundaried session, the patient can experiment with various pressures and positions of their hand in connection with the therapist's hand. A detailed example of this is presented in Chapter 8.

References

Bacal, H. A. (2011). *The power of specificity in psychotherapy: When therapy works and when it doesn't*. Jason Aronson.

Bollas, C. (2103). *Catch them before they fall: The psychoanalysis of breakdown*. Routledge. doi:10.4324/9780203069547.

Chapter 5

Brief Embodied Therapy

I believe most embodied work in psychoanalytic psychotherapy occurs in what I refer to as *brief embodied therapy*. This generally consists of 1 to 12 sessions and usually involves the first three categories of touch: pass-bys, completion touch, and some containing–informing. It typically focuses on symptom relief, such as reducing anxiety connected to trauma and specific embodied triggers that contribute to embodied flashbacks. The work may contain elements of the regressive, transitional, and progressive phases but often ends when the regressive and traumatic issues around body and touch have been addressed.

Brief embodied therapy is heavily structured and limited to specific goals and objectives. The work is often planned out in advance through discussions with the patient. This includes addressing how and what parts of the body will be engaged and what specific issues the work is designed to deal with. Often the exercises have been discussed in consultation with colleagues for possible modifications for the case at hand.

One of the attractions of brief embodied therapy is the solid boundary that is created because all physical interactions are planned out and the work is heavily structured, thus providing a built-in limit as to how far the work will proceed. If the patient or therapist starts to feel pulled into taking the work further, the preestablished frame can act as a form of anchor, keeping the work limited to the agreed on activity. Frequently, an exercise will be repeated over the course of several sessions, thereby leading to further insights and a decrease in the activation of embodied flashbacks. These exercises are processed by the patient and therapist and perhaps also in the therapist's consultation/supervision. Over time, if both patient and therapist find that the patient could benefit from continued embodied treatment, they may agree to then expand the work into other categories, such as somatic mastery and modulation and body analysis. Conversely, if through their processing they decide not to move beyond brief embodied therapy, the work can remain confined within its specific goals and objectives. This progression is another way to ensure embodied therapy remains informed and disciplined.

An example of such a situation would be a therapist working with a man who endured childhood physical abuse by his father, the experience of which

DOI: 10.4324/9781003215745-6

is reactivated whenever someone grabs his arm. As a child, the father would grab his son by the arm and drag him to his den where he beat him horrifically. In their work, this patient and his therapist agree to specifically address only his reaction to his arm being grabbed and held. The patient and therapist plan out where the work will take place, for example, in chairs, on the couch, standing, or sitting on the floor. They also consider the best way for the therapist to hold the patient's arm, such as whether it would be better to start with an open hand and then when the patient is comfortable move to more of a holding of his arm. In addition, they discuss whether and how the patient will touch the therapist: perhaps a hand on the therapist's shoulder that helps the patient feel he can push back against the therapist and feel his own adult power rather than feeling like the helpless child he had been during the beatings. Maybe the patient will also hold the therapist's arm, and the therapist can follow the patient's lead, mirroring the different pressures and grips the patient applies during the activity. They can also explore the patient's expectations for the activity, what they hope to gain from the exercise, and what they want to avoid.

An important element in this form of treatment is that prior to engaging in the work, the patient has been in talk therapy for a period of time so that the patient has become more comfortable addressing their trauma and the therapist has developed a solid understanding of the patient's traumas. When the time for engagement in brief embodied therapy arrives, the work has moved beyond a "let's try this and see what happens" mode, and the patient has had time to explore with the therapist the possibility of moving into embodied therapy.

A patient's decisions around how deeply to engage or not to engage in embodied work is similar to their decision about engaging in talk therapy. Generally, a patient who begins a psychoanalytic psychotherapy is unsure how long they will want or need to engage in treatment. Some patients decide for multiple reasons to end after only a few initial assessment sessions. Others choose to work on stated goals and objectives, and when they have achieved enough benefit, decide to end treatment. Other patients choose to move beyond specific goals and objectives into an expansive psychoanalytic psychotherapy that emphasizes addressing deeper levels of personality and character style.

Embodied treatment follows a similar pattern. The patient may decide that after beginning embodied therapy, it is not for them and request a return to talk therapy only. Others are pleased with the results of brief embodied therapy and decide to successfully end it. Others choose to move from brief embodied therapy into somatic mastery and modulation and body analysis, shifting into a more defined regressive–transitional–progressive treatment model.

Brief embodied therapy is an important modality because it offers a way to work with specific parts of embodied trauma that is an alternative to an all-

or-nothing approach. Some patients and some therapists may be more comfortable working with a specific body issue resulting from trauma rather than a fuller immersion into multiple physical issues that may feel overwhelming and even intolerable.

I do not privilege either brief or longer-term embodied therapy because both can be effective and transformative. Often, the decision of how to work with the body in treatment is less about trauma and more about the comfort level of both patient and therapist in working body to body. The issues of therapeutic fit as theorized in psychoanalysis by Bacal (2011) is found in both talk and body therapies. At times, the therapeutic fit might be optimal for talk therapy but not so much for embodied treatment. For example, gender differences between patient and therapist that are less an issue in talk therapy may become more pronounced in embodied therapy. It is also possible that the therapist's style of physical engagement does not harmonize with the patient's therapeutic needs in embodied treatment. This can be seen in massage therapy when, for example, a client wants a Swedish-style massage with gentle touch, and the massage therapist primarily does deep tissue work.

I have worked with many patients, especially women who were sexually abused, who found brief embodied therapy with me to be effective and the limit of what they were comfortable engaging with in treatment. In many such instances, they also found a female massage therapist to continue the work of reclaiming their body. They then brought their work from the massage experience back to their analysis with me, and we would integrate that work into our sessions.

In my own personal experience, I have hired and worked with many massage therapists who were good at massage but for certain reasons we could not create the therapeutic fit I needed for embodied treatment. In my first years of treatment, I needed to focus on my early childhood trauma. During that more regressive phase, I was less likely to work with someone who could not relate to my body in a regressed manner that created embodied connections with my traumatized child self-states. Later I needed a more progressive fit. If someone had difficulty relating to me and my body as an adult male and instead worked within a regressive approach, that became less effective for me. I no longer needed a primarily regressive experience but to experience my adult body. For me, the combination of regressive, transitional, and progressive work was achieved by seeking out different massage and bodywork specialists at different times. I never found one person who could move through all the phases with me. I came to understand that each massage therapist provided me with a section of work that could be added to the overall foundation of my embodied transformation. I was also able to theorize how my work with each massage therapist had been a form of brief but effective treatment for a specific embodied issue.

Thus, the specific issue or issues addressed in brief embodied therapy are not always clear-cut or precise. In addition, brief should not be confused with superficial. Although the work may address one specific form of touch that activates an embodied trauma, often brief embodied therapy addresses a deep fear or anxiety around all forms of touch. The fear of all forms of touch turning sexually or physically abusive was the issue addressed in brief embodied therapy with a patient I have written about before, whom I call Charlotte (see Novak, 2018).

My Work with Charlotte

I suspected from the beginning of Charlotte's treatment that therapeutic touch might be helpful. However, I did not think I would be able to offer it to her, given her overt comments about wanting to have sex with me. This case demonstrates how, given enough time in talk therapy to establish a trusting relationship, and then working within a heavily structured brief embodied therapeutic frame, a patient may be able to make use of embodied treatment and begin the long but enlivening journey of recovering their stolen body.

Charlotte was a young college graduate student who was attending therapy for issues of intense anxiety and debilitating chronic pain that seemed connected to her torturous upbringing. Charlotte's father had left her mother on discovering she was pregnant with Charlotte. Her mother had not wanted Charlotte and often expressed her hatred for Charlotte through verbal, physical, and sexual abuse. Her mother's physical beatings left marks on Charlotte's arms and legs, and she was instructed to lie when questioned by school counselors to say the bruises were the result of playground mishaps. Her mother's sexual touch was explained as "love," and given how badly her mother treated Charlotte and despite feeling uncomfortable and confused by the sexual touching, it was the only time Charlotte felt anything close to love from her mother or anyone else. In addition to her own sexual abuse of Charlotte, in exchange for money her mother made Charlotte available to men who sexually abused her in what seemed to have been an undercover sex ring.

At age 17, Charlotte left home for college and graduated with a business degree. She began working with me when she was in her mid-twenties and engaged in a successful business career. However, she continued to struggle with relational and emotional issues from her years of childhood abuse and was now coming to terms with what she had labeled "love" in childhood actually being sexual abuse. This realization, along with visual and somatic flashbacks, made it hard for her to enjoy her adult life. Charlotte used alcohol and marijuana heavily to self-medicate and manage daily embodied trauma flashbacks.

Although Charlotte's embodied traumas had created both intimacy issues around physical engagement and health issues, I decided that I would not introduce the possibility of embodied therapy. My reasoning was that, given her childhood had been saturated with chronic and severe physical and sexual abuse, physical interactions with me in treatment might be too confusing for her. I was not sure if she would be able to experience my motivations as therapeutic rather than as another form of exploitation designed to eventually lead to sexual encounters. In addition, Charlotte's abuse had created in her a more hypersexualized relationship to physical contact. I thought perhaps any embodied therapy might be sexualized by her. She had grown up seeing, as she said, "My body and me being only good for one thing: sex."

Prior to working with Charlotte, I had only been comfortable working with patients whose sexual abuse had resulted in an avoidance of sex. Using touch with patients who sexualized all touch seemed too risky, and my own skills and abilities in embodied therapy had reached my personal limit. I would either need to accept this limit and not use embodied treatment with patients who had hypersexual responses to sexual abuse or expand my understanding of embodied work. As I said at the start of this chapter, I had already decided, well before I met Charlotte, that this embodied work was beyond my level of comfort and ability. However, Charlotte's commitment to treatment, her desire to recover her stolen body, and her need to find some relief from her chronic pain made me rethink my position as we worked on her issues and developed a solid therapeutic relationship. Ultimately, our work together in embodied treatment would provide me with a new perspective on working with hypersexual responses to sexual abuse.

In many sessions during the first year of therapy, Charlotte talked about sexual thoughts she had about me during the week and even in session. She said that these occurred "because the only way I know how to relate to men is through sex." These were not primarily sexual fantasies but rather habitual thoughts that were quite common for her relative to men. I never felt Charlotte attempting to seduce me. Rather, her sexualization of our relationship felt like something she did with every man who paid attention to her. Relating in a sexualized manner was what she thought was required of her. My way of processing this with her therapeutically was the beginning of her trusting my responses would be therapeutic rather than sexual. This new experience helped to establish the type of safe and sacred space required for embodied therapy.

Over the first year of our work, physical interaction was limited to a brief handshake at the end of a session. I would describe these as a blend of pass-by, completion touch, and informing touch because she was curious about what physical contact with me might feel like. Sometimes, rather than a session-ending handshake, Charlotte would ask for a hug. These requests initially felt flirtatious but in a more mischievous way as opposed to a more genuine adult seduction. At least that was how I felt as I experienced her as a young college coed and myself as a middle-aged man. I also think Charlotte already knew my answer would be "no" before she even asked, given the respectful smirk on her face when I explained I would not hug her. Usually, I attempted to match her mischievous request with my own playful smile and response so as not to shame her or have her feel criticized or judged. I generally said something like, "You just spent the session talking about wanting to have sex with me on my couch, and now you think I'm going to be comfortable with us hugging?" My raised eyebrows and smile were always met with a smile and laughter from Charlotte.

In these instances, I did offer a handshake for multiple reasons. One was that the sessions were intense, with Charlotte working hard on her traumas and discovering repressed and dissociated memories of abuse and the accompanying intolerable emotions and body sensations. The handshakes were a less confusing form of completion touch and a source of connection for her.

As her therapy continued, Charlotte began to have fewer thoughts of acting out with me sexually and became more focused on her horrific childhood abuse and neglect. She continued to discover many ways in which her traumas had poisoned her relationship with her body. She was able to speak of how genuine bodily pleasure, both sexual and nonsexual, seemed elusive. She was also deepening her understanding of how her physical relationships with both men and women were confusing and limited because any forms of physical comfort had the potential to activate her childhood traumas. She began to understand how her body had been used as a sex object, and because that had been the only form of attention she received, that was how she related even now. She was, for the first time, beginning to understand that her abuse was not normal and not her fault. She was developing kindness toward herself, especially toward her child self-state that included mourning her lost childhood.

Here is an illustration of how the brief embodied therapy work around engaging in handshakes, processing, and consulting about them helped inform my decision about if and when to engage in a therapeutic hug with Charlotte.

As our work together continued, issues around Charlotte's childhood traumas intensified. Occasionally, at the end of a session she talked about wanting a hug but being anxious about getting one. However, over time, when she extended her hand for our completion touch handshake, she now seemed genuinely disappointed with that ending and perhaps disappointed with me not offering a hug. I felt her motivation for a hug at that point was different from the previous mischievous requests, and her sexualization of me had decreased significantly, making a therapeutic hug more possible. In addition, the end-of-session handshakes were becoming less of a pass-by. Rather than deliberate and quick as they had been, they were becoming softer and longer in duration, with brief but meaningful eye contact, a solid form of completion touch. In consultations, I began discussing the possible therapeutic benefits and potential confusion a hug at the end of a session might create for Charlotte. I used our recent therapy and handshakes, my consultations, and the sense that the hug seemed to be connected to her trauma work to inform my decision whether and when to agree to a hug.

I certainly was not surprised and was now actually prepared for Charlotte's revisiting her request for a session-ending hug. I too had been feeling close to her in the context of her trauma work and even a bit parental. In those months, Charlotte had become more aware of her transference toward me as a caring parental figure.

One day, while facing me at the end of a session, instead of extending her hand for a handshake, Charlotte apprehensively asked if she could have a hug. With genuine curiosity, I said, "This request feels different to me." She agreed and said that she felt the way she did when she wanted a hug as a child. This brief processing was the final piece of information I needed to inform my decision and agree to the hug.

The hug, a form of completion touch, was brief but also informative. For 5 seconds, Charlotte wrapped her arms around me and buried her head into my chest. I was surprised by this intense response, and I think Charlotte was too because I had barely placed my arms around her when the brief moment of her melting into my arms and relaxing ended by her pushing me away and saying, "No, I can't want this!" and quickly leaving.

We processed this hug in the following session. Charlotte said she noticed both a strong desire and fear in wanting to hug me. She feared her desire was sexual, despite not noticing any sexual feelings. I too did not experience her hug, or mine, as sexual. She had feared, despite knowing this fear was from her childhood abuse, that I would turn on her and begin physically abusing and punching her. I found it informative that she was more worried about me physically harming her than fearing I would turn the hug into something sexual. Perhaps she trusted she was safe sexually but not physically. She said she was "pretty sure" I would not punch her like her mom had. She described how her mother would engage in a sadistic game in which she would offer affection, such as a hug, but then slap or punch her. Charlotte's internal struggle between a desire for physical comfort while at the same time being terrified of it was heartbreaking. Something so important and meaningful in life, physical contact, was suspicious and terrifying.

For the next 2 months there was no physical engagement or completion touch at the end of the sessions because Charlotte seemed to need time to process her fears of me, and others, relative to touch. My consultations affirmed that any continued embodied work would need to proceed slowly and at Charlotte's pace. Following consultations, rather than continuing with any physical contact, I decided to focus the embodied work on helping Charlotte explore ways she could self-soothe. This produced limited results. I guided her in deep-breathing exercises, using her hands and arms to self-embrace, and touching her own face and hair. However, Charlotte could not make use of these self-soothing behaviors.

As discussed in Chapter 1, I find this often to be the case for individuals with trauma histories. Many patients who were abused never had comforting or soothing touch following the abuse. They were left alone to deal with its effects, which is a monumental undertaking for a child. A necessary ingredient of repair from trauma—an embodied connection with an empathic other—was missing. In therapy, when they attempt to work on ways to self-soothe during trauma flashbacks, there are few if any experiences of embodied comfort from primary caregivers to draw from. Thus, usually there are limits to how much self-soothing can be achieved relative to embodied trauma.

I continued to work with Charlotte as both new and more detailed memories became available to her. She brought these to session and we processed them together. During this period of two sessions per week, Charlotte's marijuana and alcohol use grew as a way of finding relief from the intense emotions and body sensations that increased as more and clearer memories of her childhood surfaced.

One Monday she arrived for her session high, saying she had been "drinking and smoking weed all weekend." Her anxiety was even more intense than usual, and she found substance use to be the only way to reduce it. At the end of the session I requested that she try to arrive for her next scheduled session (on Thursday) sober. I was considering revisiting physical contact, and I believed an absence of empathic embodied connection with me was, in some ways, reenacting the original trauma in which comfort contact was unavailable. I needed her to be sober in order for me to feel confident processing the possibility of making use of touch to provide a form of embodied connection within her trauma memories. Again, I felt that, given the profound absence of healthy touch and physical comfort in her life, I was going to have to provide this experience for her and help her to make use of it.

Charlotte arrived on Thursday sober and noticeably anxious. She began pacing and saying, "I'd be OK if this damn little girl in me would just shut up and go away." Knowing this was how her mother spoke and related to her, I responded with, "How did your mother get in here?" My response evoked a smile, a deep exhale, and a slight reduction in her anxiety. She sat down, and I shared my thoughts that perhaps it was time for us to revisit touch in her treatment as a way to help her to manage her anxiety. I explained my thinking and asked if sitting next to one another on the couch would be OK. She agreed, and we sat next to each other for a while without any contact. She described feeling both a little calmer and at the same time more aware of some of the fears associated with her childhood abuse.

We spent 20 minutes talking and processing these responses until there was enough clarity and agreement that continuing the work with her body would be beneficial. With her permission, I leaned slightly closer so that our shoulders made mild contact. This was a form of containing–informing contact—more informing than containing as evidenced by her comment: "This feels weird." She explained that she noticed that my body did not feel either "sexual" or "angry," just "calm and relaxed." She was correct: My body felt relaxed and welcoming. However, Charlotte did not know how to experience or make use of this form of empathic physical closeness.

In addition, even though my body felt relaxed to her, she worried that her feelings about our physical contact were being sexualized by her. She told me that she was not thinking or wanting to relate to me sexually but that "it's just what my body expects." As she sat and thought more, she noted that although her body was feeling some involuntary excitement she did not want to act on the feelings. In that moment, she recognized her ability to contain her feelings and control her behavioral responses. This was important because she was becoming more confident that she was able to trust not only me to hold the boundary but herself as well.

Because she could now trust the boundary on both sides, Charlotte was able to be more curious about our embodied connection. She noticed that the sensation of our shoulders touching helped her to feel a little less anxious. As her therapist, I could sense her body relaxing and her breathing became calmer and deeper. She was speaking less and was internally reflective. She said she was noticing and experiencing our physical contact as comforting rather than sexually or physically abusive.

In our following Monday session, Charlotte reported being sober all weekend, ever since Thursday. She believed our physical contact had acted as a model for soothing and that maybe she could now learn how to self-soothe. It was not until after the session that it dawned on me that we had not used any touch in the session because we had spent most of the time processing the touch from the previous week.

That Thursday, Charlotte began by telling me about her week. I did not pay much attention to her moving the cushions on the couch until she gently, and with a smile, patted the space she had made there for me so I could sit next to her. I asked if she wanted me to move there, and she smiled and nodded. I did not experience her request as sexual, seductive, or even flirtatious. My internal reaction to her request was similar to a parent being asked by a child. I certainly was aware that Charlotte was a woman and not a child, but at that moment there was a sense of playful innocence about her. However, before I moved to the couch, I inquired about why she had not asked for any touch in the previous session. I wanted to make sure I was assessing the moment accurately. Charlotte said that she had wanted to ask me to sit next to her but was afraid that I would say no or make fun of her, just as her mother had done. Charlotte was able to compare her fears of shame and rejection to this new and uncomfortable but relieving response of acceptance and being taken seriously by me. Following this conversation, I moved over to the space she had created for me on the couch.

After I moved to the couch, Charlotte leaned over and initiated contact with my shoulder and arm with hers. She could only tolerate 1 or 2 minutes of touch before needing to stand up and walk around the room as she processed the experience. We repeated this exercise several times in the session. At one point, I made the mistake of touching her forearm with my hand, and she rose abruptly from the couch and walked around. I had moved too fast by doing something that had not been introduced so that Charlotte could anticipate it. My move off of the planned, structured activity into a spontaneous gesture was something that Charlotte was not ready to receive. Although my sponta-neous gesture seemed to be mild, for many patients with abuse histories, the issue is not the type of touch but the fact that they were unable to anticipate the con-tact. I apologized and we processed my mistake.

Charlotte said my hand on her forearm had felt good but that like some of our previous work, that form of therapeutic touch was still foreign to her. She was still becoming used to physical touch not turning sexual or abusive. She was also able to make an important link between my spontaneously touching her forearm and her childhood traumas. She now remembered how her mother would often hold her hand and then painfully twist it. She believed the embodied trauma memory of her mother's sadistic arm twisting was triggered when I touched her forearm. Charlotte added that a relaxed hand like mine was something she had never experienced in childhood, and, as an adult, she was used to either no touch or sexualized touch. It appeared con-tact comfort touch as a child had been either infrequent or, she guessed, never available.

Our sessions began to include touch, shoulder to shoulder, and eventually brief hand holding. These forms of touch were a mixture of contact comfort and containing–informing. We also used completion touch in the form of a hug at the end of the session. These completion touch hugs occurred approximately once or twice a month, always at her request. In that phase of the treatment, I always agreed to the hug.

Over time, Charlotte began to trust that a request for contact comfort touch was not going to end in physical abuse, turn sexual, or be made fun of. This included her own increased capacity to trust that she could hold a ther-apeutic boundary as well. This transferred to relationships outside of therapy as she felt more confident in her abilities to hold healthy boundaries with other men. She noticed that her ability to engage in various forms of non-sexual touch with others was increasing, and her somatic symptoms continued to slowly but significantly reduce. She said that she had even engaged in a few nonsexual hugs with friends between sessions and that they felt "strange but comforting."

The brief embodied therapy with Charlotte occurred for eight sessions. However, completion touch hugs and handshakes remained part of her treat-ment throughout the remainder of her therapy with me. Charlotte and I did not seem to be in a position to work any further with physical contact at that point in her treatment. Perhaps we had even hit a limit in the therapeutic fit where, for her, embodied therapy with an older man might be too anxiety provoking, given her sexual abuse in childhood. Her issues of sexual abuse and physical torture were too deep and severe to make work beyond contact comfort, completion, and containing–informing forms of touch safe and therapeutic with me. At that point, further embodied therapy most likely would have been quite confusing and unsettling for her and perhaps even beyond my ability to effectively execute. More years of talk therapy would have been required to develop the therapeutic connection required for working in the more expansive forms of embodied therapy that are found in somatic mastery and modulation and body analysis.

Charlotte ended her therapy with me approximately a year after the brief embodied work just described. Throughout the final year of our work, the only use of physical contact was occasional completion touch at the end of a session in the form of a handshake or hug. However, the brief embodied therapy continued to inform her work in traditional psychoanalytic psychotherapy without touch. She often described the ways in which that work had impacted her relationship with her own body. She also talked about her improved capacity to engage physically with others in ways that were not exclusively sexualized.

Certainly Charlotte and I both recognized that the types of trauma and torture she endured as a child were issues that could not be fully resolved in the therapy she did with me and that she still had work ahead of her. However, the brief embodied treatment and our continued use of handshakes and hugs were an important step in her reclaiming her stolen body.

References

Bacal, H. A. (2011). *The power of specificity in psychotherapy: When therapy works and when it doesn't*. Jason Aronson.

Novak, E. T. (2018). A model of informed physical contact in psychotherapy. *Transactional Analysis Journal*, 48(1), 18–32. doi:10.1080/03621537.2018.1397962.

Chapter 6

Embodied Misattunements and Mistakes that Are Part of Treatment and Boundary Violations that Are Not

My main focus in this chapter is how to distinguish between misattunements and mistakes in embodied psychotherapy and how to process and work through them. The fear of making a mistake when doing this kind of work always comes up in my presentations and discussions with colleagues. This chapter will explain and then demonstrate with a case vignette how misattunements and mistakes are a normal and expected part of any embodied treatment and how boundary violations are a separate issue that falls outside of any ethical therapeutic treatment.

One problem facing the therapist when working directly with the patient's body in therapy is that our profession provides few examples of how to process and proceed during and following an embodied treatment misattunement or mistake. In psychoanalysis, the term *enactment* (Jacobs, 1986) describes moments and events in treatment in which both patient and therapist can have unconscious or unknown parts of themselves activated. For those familiar with the construct of enactment, what I am describing in this section could often, but not always, be viewed as a form of embodied enactment. However, I will not use that analytic word, preferring the terms *misattunements* and *mistakes*.

The disruption to the therapist can be more intense if they fear the embodied misattunement or mistake might be erroneously framed as an ethical boundary violation rather than as a common situation in embodied trauma work that needs to be processed and worked through. Contributing to the therapist's anxiety is the profession's ingrained suspicion of touch and the corresponding lack of theory and published clinical examples of this process, including mistakes, in psychoanalytic psychotherapy. As a result, there are limited professional resources available about how to address embodied misattunements or mistakes.

This is a good time to remind the reader that patients who want to do embodied therapy are highly motivated. They are committing to working in ways they know will evoke multiple reactions—pleasant, unpleasant, sometimes even unbearable—in order to reclaim their bodies. The patient's focus is on the possibility of discovering and recovering their stolen body both

DOI: 10.4324/9781003215745-7

independently of and in relationship to others. Generally, their fears and anxieties are more about moving into treatment that is directly focused on their body rather than possible mistakes made by their trusted therapist, someone by that point they have known for years. Often, the possibility of embodied change and transformation seems daunting, and patients can become upset or angry when either a misattunement or mistake occurs. However, they generally are willing and want to process, understand, and make use of such moments in order to adjust the treatment and move deeper into their important work. Another reminder is that embodied therapy should only begin after both patient and therapist have developed a level of mutual trust and an understanding of the patient's therapeutic needs relative to embodied therapy.

As those who have done their own intensive psychoanalytic psychotherapy know, the road to transformation is not smooth or easy, especially when addressing trauma. Misattunements and mistakes often create ruptures in the therapeutic relationship that the patient and therapist then need to process and repair, sometimes over several sessions. This is a common component of psychoanalytic psychotherapy and can be intense and difficult. However, it can also lead to a deeper understanding and connection. The same is true of misattunements and mistakes during embodied therapy. Distinguishing between a misattunement and a mistake is difficult because there are no clear distinctions between them and there can be some overlap.

Embodied Misattunements

In embodied therapy, misattunements occur when the form of embodied connection is slightly different from or out of sync with what the patient is anticipating or wanting at that moment within a specific self-state experience. For example, a therapist might offer a firm hand squeeze when the patient would prefer lighter pressure because they are trying to remain within a more intrapsychic space. The firmer pressure, designed to create a more solid connection, creates a distraction. I find Winnicott's (1965) use of the word "impingement" (p. 34) useful. Unlike a more complementary embodied connection that enhances the patient's ability to explore a specific self-state, an impingement interrupts or intrudes on the patient's deeper immersion into that self-state.

A misattunement or impingement is generally experienced by the patient as the therapist being with them in their current self-state experience but not fully attuned within the physical connection. Nonetheless, the patient may still be able to tolerate and make use of a slight misattunement. Processing misattunements helps the therapist understand the patient's needs in those moments and to make appropriate adjustments. The processing and reworking of specific embodied connections is one of the ways both patient and therapist can develop the type of implicit embodied connections required for deeper work in somatic mastery and modulation and body analysis.

Readers who engage in massage may be aware of misattunements that can occur in that context. For example, the massotherapist may use too much pressure when the client is trying to move into a relaxed space. The client may have to ask the massotherapist to ease up. I have also heard from many patients that they felt too uncomfortable to tell their massotherapist that the pressure was either too hard or too gentle or that they wanted to have more attention paid to a specific body area. That is unfortunate, because the massotherapist usually wants to know.

In embodied therapy, patients may be equally reluctant to tell the therapist when something is not working for them. I have had patients wait several sessions before they could, apprehensively, ask me if we could adjust part of the embodied work. Sometimes they want less touch, such as moving from sitting beside one another to sitting chair to chair. At other times they want a different kind of touch, such as stroking their hair or massaging their feet or arms. In processing these feelings, they are often afraid that I will mockingly reject their request as inappropriate. That has never been my experience of their request. In exploring such situations, the patient slowly begins to claim a healthy sense that they no longer have to tolerate physical misattunements but can assertively address them. In addition, if for some reason I find I am not confident in the therapeutic benefits of their request, or have reached my own limitations, then exploring alternative forms of touch can also signal to the patient that their request is being taken seriously rather than being judged as inappropriate or strange.

Embodied Mistakes

I distinguish between two types of mistakes in embodied therapy: *procedural* and *clinical*. Procedural mistakes involve using touch when the patient is ambivalent about incorporating it into the treatment or the therapy has not developed to the point at which embodied therapy is appropriate. An example might be engaging in touch too soon, such as hugging a patient without having talked about such a possibility beforehand. Two of the most common procedural mistakes are moving too quickly into touch or using advanced forms of embodied therapy prematurely.

Clinical embodied mistakes are similar to misattunements. These occur when the type of touch being used does not match the type needed by the patient in that moment, but, unlike misattunements, the patient cannot make use of the physical connection. In such instances, the patient experiences the physical interaction as incongruent with the self-state they are in. Clinical mistakes can intensify an embodied trauma memory or embodied flashback. For example, when a patient is in a regressive trauma memory and the therapist uses forms of touch that are better suited to either the transitional or progressive phase of treatment. Clinical mistakes occur more often with patients who have experienced multiple embodied traumas at different times in their lives. A form of physical connection that works well with one self-state can be a trauma trigger in another self-state.

There are examples of clinical mistakes in the cases described in Chapters 7 through 10. In those treatments, both patients had experienced multiple traumas at different ages, and I made clinical mistakes regarding the physical connection I offered.

Mistakes are also more common both early in embodied treatment and when using the first three categories of touch (pass-bys, completion touch, and containing–informing touch), likely because both patient and therapist are still learning how to engage with one another at an embodied level. In addition, the therapist is still learning what forms of touch may activate the patient's trauma. Often even the patient is unaware that a particular movement or contact can activate a specific embodied trauma.

By the time the work progresses into somatic mastery and modulation and body analysis, both patient and therapist are attuned to each other's bodies and can anticipate ways of moving and relating physically. At that point, incongruencies can more often be categorized as misattunements or impingements, with the correction occurring "on the fly" in that moment in the session and processing happening later.

Generally, with patients, I am more likely to use the term mistake rather than misattunement because many traumatized individuals were told by their abuser that the abuse was their fault. In addition, many abusers blame themselves for their abuse. I have found, especially early in trauma work, that trying to process a physical interaction that disrupts or overwhelms the patient by talking about it as something that was cocreated or as a misattunement tends to intensify the disruption. That is because the patient can interpret what I am saying as either blaming them, minimizing the experience, or not taking ownership of my contribution in causing the disruption.

When my physical engagement with a patient evokes an embodied flashback for them, my own feelings of self-criticism can be a powerful motivator for me to minimize or repair a mistake too quickly. Sometimes I am in a hurry to repair in order to reduce my own guilt and anxiety for having activated a patient's embodied flashback. My attempts to explain, justify, or quickly repair my mistake rather than stay with the patient's experience of how it may have evoked elements of their original trauma usually only worsens the situation. My explanations are often received as me saying, "I didn't do anything wrong." The patient often hears my words as a form of "I didn't want that—you did," "You made me do it," "It is your fault," and other forms of blame that sound similar to what their abuser said.

I find that genuinely admitting my mistake followed by processing the patient's reaction to it can be powerful. Most people who were abused or neglected never receive a meaningful apology or admission of guilt from their abuser. My genuine apology also implicitly signals that I "own" my therapeutic mistake, which is in stark contrast to how their abuser may have denied the abuse or even blamed them for it. If a patient is angry at me for activating an embodied flashback, I stay with their anger before moving into an apology and repair. Many patients never could be overtly angry at their abuser, and it is an important part of their work to be able to express anger without retaliation from their therapist.

For the therapist to process a mistake in this way, they must remain confident that it occurred within a therapeutic frame as part of the process of embodied work rather than fearing accusations of wrongdoing, even when the patient may be confused in the moment about the therapist's intent. This is not much different from a mistake or rupture in talk therapy but, because the work is physical, the therapist's anxiety may be even more intense. However, by the time the patient and therapist are engaged in this physical work, there should already be a level of trust established on both sides such that the idea of wrongdoing, ulterior motives, or exploitation would be rooted primarily within the patient's past traumas rather than the motivations of a good therapist.

Processing a mistake or misattunement becomes easier as patient and therapist become familiar with how to process physical interactions with one another. In fact, if there is a concern on either side that being able to process the work is not yet possible, then physical work should not be started.

I have also found that, given the intensity of embodied work, a mutual exchange between patient and therapist about what is working and what is not is essential. The patient needs to know and believe that anything they are uncomfortable with can and should be brought to the therapist's attention. A patient should never tolerate embodied work because, for whatever reason, they feel that they cannot speak up. Following processing, the patient may decide they do want to tolerate the fear or discomfort created by a form of touch in order to work through an embodied trauma memory. However, this is different from the patient tolerating something without the therapist's awareness or without a mutual understanding of why the patient wants to stay with the discomfort.

Boundary Violations and Patient Exploitation

Mistakes and misattunements stand in contrast to boundary violations, most of which involve physical contact that is either unwelcome, not a part of a treatment agreement, or created through manipulation of the patient (including the therapist's misuse of their position of power). In such instances, the therapist's motivation for touch is for their own gratification (usually but not always sexual). It has little or nothing to do with therapeutic work and is a deliberate exploitation of the patient. As we know, many boundary violations occur in therapies that do not even use embodied approaches.

My father used to say, "Eddie, car locks only keep honest people out of your car." Like car locks, codes of ethics are helpful for professionals who are committed to high standards of treatment but do not prevent therapists with malicious intent from abusing or exploiting patients. Boundary violations, psychological manipulations, abuse, and exploitation of patients by therapists can occur in both typical talk therapy and embodied psychotherapy. I cannot emphasize strongly enough that ethical psychoanalytic psychotherapy and embodied therapy require that the therapist not treat the patient's body as a tool for the therapist's own sexual or other narcissistic gratification. Sadly, I have worked with many patients who have experienced boundary violations or were exploited in other ways by previous therapists. Sometimes this has even occurred under the guise of "bodywork."

A boundary violation can also occur not out of conscious, malicious intent but unintentionally as the result of the therapist not having done enough of their own work and study or obtaining enough clinical consultation to ensure the work remains within therapeutic boundaries. A therapist's in-depth exploration of their own body and mind, as well as clinical consultations, are crucial for reducing the risks of unintentional boundary violations.

In addition, ethical embodied work that is solidly anchored in theory, a clear framework, and agreed-on contracts can help keep the work safe and less confusing for the patient. Again, major safeguards include the therapist's understanding of multiple theories, the use of case consultation, and engaging in personal embodied therapy.

In ethical embodied therapy, boundary issues are not primarily about actual touch but rather about what the touch means for the patient. This is because each patient has a different history and experience of touch. However, I have found in consultation with many therapists that they are looking for reassurance that they did not do anything ethically wrong by touching their patient. Nevertheless, many forms of physical engagement that do not involve a boundary violation can still create discomfort or confusion for a patient. The focus needs to move beyond the physical touch and include a detailed exploration of the patient's response and the unique meaning of the touch for them.

Exploring the unique meaning of physical touch is essential in all forms of embodied interactions in treatment, not just when there is confusion about it. If the embodied psychotherapy is guided and anchored in theory, frame, and contract, boundary violations are no more likely to occur than in typically talk-only psychotherapy. When a therapist is working theoretically, engaged in consultation, and has extensive experience in their own bodywork, they should not be overly focused on fear of ethical violations. When a form of physical contact feels uncomfortable, confusing, or even exploitive, especially within a traumatized self-state, it is important for the therapist to be empathic and open to exploring such instances rather than defensively justifying any touch that felt uncomfortable to the patient.

One of the most important elements in maintaining healthy boundaries is the patient's and therapist's understanding and respect for the sacredness of the body in embodied therapy. In psychoanalytic psychotherapy there are times when a patient is working within deep parts of the self that require, by their nature, deep connection with and commitment from their therapist. Embodied work requires this same level of commitment and an ethos that recognizes the sacredness of working within the terrain of a stolen body. In the space of embodied therapeutic relatedness there is a profound respect for the body that is inviolable. This sacredness goes beyond ethics and demands a therapeutic reverence for the embodied vulnerability of the patient.

I end this chapter with a case vignette that describes some procedural mistakes I made early in my career. These were primarily the result of my still-limited understanding of embodied therapy and moving too quickly into embodied work. I believe this example reflects a common way that well-intentioned therapists make mistakes with touch in the clinical setting.

The Case on the Couch

This composite case reflects mistakes I made with a few patients and many of the factors that contributed to these mistakes. I then speculate on how other mistakes or even possible boundary violations can occur in similar situations in an embodied treatment that is premature or conducted without a systematic process or knowledge of how to work in embodied therapy.

A woman who learned I had experience working with embodied trauma contacted me for treatment. In our first session, she said that she believed physical contact, specifically holding my hand, would make it easier for her to speak about her issues. She was a few years older than me, with children similar in age to my son, so there seemed to be a connection around many issues, including parenting. I think these commonalities, her stated curiosity about embodied work, my skills being limited to simple body exercises rather than embodied therapy, and my overly enthusiastic desire to work with patients at an embodied level all contributed to my moving much too quickly into a poorly informed and poorly disciplined physical engagement with her.

I did know to begin slowly, but I did not work slowly enough. I was not curious enough about her motivations or my overeagerness in wanting to make use of embodied work. One of my first mistakes had to do with us not knowing one another well enough. The therapy was just beginning, and a true therapeutic relationship was not yet established enough to begin intense trauma work within talk therapy, let alone venturing into embodied work. I certainly did not know her or her traumas well enough to proceed at the pace and categories of touch into which we moved.

In the second session, she asked if she could hold my hand while sitting next to me on the couch. I was uncomfortable with that arrangement, and I offered instead to move my two large office chairs together. This was at least a slow beginning to embodied work, even if we were beginning the work prematurely. As I mentioned in Chapter 4, sitting next to a patient in chairs is a way I often begin embodied treatment with patients. I find the chairs help provide a built-in physical boundary.

The embodied work began with the patient and I holding hands while sitting in the chairs. A mistake that the reader may notice here is that there was no processing of this beforehand. At that time in my training, I had experienced some bodywork, but I really had no idea how to prepare a patient and myself for the work. It took on too much of the "let's try this and see what happens" flavor that I warned about in Chapter 5. In addition, I naively trusted that the patient knew what she needed relative to embodied work. Instead, I should have helped her be more curious about what she was expecting, which would have also been more informative for me.

We sat holding hands, and the patient said this was helping her speak more freely. We continued in this way for two more weekly sessions when she stated during the fifth session that this form of contact did not feel like enough. She said again that what she really needed was for us to sit on the couch together. Today, after 30 years of working with the body, I would not make this mistake. However, back then I had many things to learn about embodied therapy, one of the most important being to always stick to the original plan. Especially early in treatment, if any changes are to be made, they should be about moving backward from the original plan, not forward, unless a thorough processing indicates otherwise. Sitting on the couch together with my patient was beyond what we had initially agreed to and should have been discussed more both with her and in consultation. In fact, when I consult with other therapists on their embodied work with a patient, I often find the absence of detailed processing or consultation before a movement forward to be a common error.

To return to my case, I was also ignoring my own anxiety about the move to the couch, dismissing it as being based in my own traumas rather than in my therapeutic senses. This is yet another reason the therapist needs to have addressed their own body issues. Uneasy feelings need to be explored and understood in terms of where they originate and what they might mean, often in consultation and before moving forward.

Once on the couch and holding hands, the patient's body did seem to relax more. I could sense the energy in her body shift. However, her conversation became more flirtatious with a seductive tone. In addition, I was not locating any regressive material or trauma memories in her words or body. There was no sense of anxiety in her body, but there certainly was in mine. Rather than the sense of inhibition most patients have in an initial shift in this work, the patient seemed to be overly comfortable. I began to sense I was being seduced. I was, in part, not believing it, and in another way, I was becoming terrified. My suspicions seemed confirmed when she asked if she could lay down and put her head in my lap. This is how quickly things can escalate within the work without proper planning, discussions, understanding, and a model. I now had myself, and the patient, moving into a potentially compromising situation.

Fortunately, I was able to work out a therapeutic end to this mistake. I merely stated that I did not feel the move to the couch was creating the therapeutic structure I thought it would and that we needed to move back to the chairs. Notice I did not blame her, because the decision to move to the couch was ultimately my responsibility, not hers. I spoke about the treatment process and that this was a therapeutic decision based on my belief that the move to the couch was not therapeutically helpful.

Internally, I felt terrible that I had moved too fast and maybe had shamed the patient or made her feel like she had done something wrong. She had not, and she was able to respect my ownership of the mistake. However, I was so worried I had done something deeply wrong that the process note for that session read like a dissertation!

I sought consultation following the session, which helped my understanding of what had happened and how to proceed. In our next session—on the chairs, which were now separated from one another—I was able to speak to her about the move to and back from the couch and the adjustments I thought were needed in her therapy going forward. I was able to explain, based on how early we were in treatment, that continued bodywork might not be optimal, that instead we needed to slow the psychotherapy down and suspend embodied work for now. She was agreeable, and that is what we did.

Over the next 6 months, there were no more sessions with touch. We began to address many of the issues the patient had sought treatment for, both childhood trauma and current marital issues. In my talk therapy with her, I learned that seductive behavior was something she had engaged in for most of her adult life, generally without much thought. She said, "This is just what I do. I don't know why." We began to understand how her own traumas had resulted in a hypersexualized way of relating to men. If I had known then what I know now, and if bodywork had been something we reengaged in, we would have needed an approach similar to the one I used with Charlotte as described in Chapter 5. However, the treatment ended abruptly when her husband accepted a transfer and the family moved.

What makes processing these kinds of mistakes challenging is that in both psychotherapy and psychoanalysis we have yet to establish a clinical framework for embodied therapy that can be used as a guide in processing embodied mistakes. To develop such a framework, I have looked to body psychotherapy, massage therapy, and consultations with colleagues. In my processing of this case, I see my errors as primarily procedural mistakes due in part to not having an integrated theory and model of embodied therapy.

Another mistake was moving too quickly into working with embodied process. The patient's therapy had not progressed enough to begin work with touch. A therapeutic shift to the couch would have required many more sessions on the chairs and many more consultations in order to understand what was needed in the treatment. I also would have needed to experiment more with working on the couch in my own embodied work. All of that might have given me a better understanding of what the patient and I would be doing as well as what needed to happen and not happen. Today, regardless of how in tune I might be with a patient, I would not move from chairs to couch so quickly or, indeed, even to working with touch on the chairs. This case is an example of how the absence of a sound theory and model of informed touch can lead to a quick escalation of issues within an embodied situation.

In more advanced therapy, such as body analysis, a new form of touch may be added spontaneously in a session. However, even then touch should move no more than one increment forward. For example, if patient and therapist are holding hands, an incremental increase could be a squeeze of the hand, two hands holding one hand, or both hands being held. A shift to putting an arm around the patient or even a mutual embrace would extend the physical contact too far beyond the agreed on structured activity. Sometimes, embodied therapy does proceed in this more spontaneous fashion, but my concern with such a spontaneous style is that the work can get close to the "let's try it and see what happens" approach that is neither an informed nor a disciplined way of working. Generally, any new forms of touch—such as a shift from chairs to couch—are best processed before moving forward with them.

References

Jacobs, T. (1986). On countertransference and enactments. *Journal of the American Psychoanalytic Association*, 34, 289–302. doi:10.1177/000306518603400203.

Winnicott, D. W. (1965). The maturational processes and the facilitating environment: Studies in the theory of emotional development. *The International Psychoanalytical Library*, 64, 1–276. The Hogarth Press and the Institute of Psychoanalysis. doi:10.4324/9780429482410.

Chapter 7

Mike

An Integration of Psychoanalytic Psychotherapy and Embodied Therapy

Mike was in his mid-twenties when he began seeing me for traditional psychoanalytic psychotherapy. His presenting issues were generalized depression and anxiety, including panic attacks that were related to childhood abuse and traumatization. The work focused primarily on how his trauma history continued to invade and complicate his daily life and relationships.

Mike had been in several brief therapies prior to seeing me and had been diagnosed with post-traumatic stress disorder (PTSD). He described his previous therapeutic work as cognitive behavioral therapy that provided some mild and temporary relief from what he was feeling. However, those modest gains were not enough for him. He was tired of feeling anxious and depressed all of the time and wanted to try something different.

In the third year of our work together, the therapy around his childhood abuse deepened as Mike began to provide more details and experience more emotions and somatic sensations. This is not uncommon when someone moves deeper into trauma work. I was witnessing memories of his abuse through his verbal descriptions, anxiety and terror, and somatic sensations. He continued to disclose, remember, and feel even more of his traumas, especially those that had been split-off, dissociated, and never acknowledged by his parents. This included an incident when Mike was 8 and his father's physical violence escalated to choking him until Mike passed out. He believed it was possible that his father could have killed him while his mother watched and did nothing. Mike reported that his parents denied any history of this abuse when he confronted them.

Mike's embodied memories tortured him most of the day and even more intensely at night. Connected to these feelings of terror and panic were the type of paranoid thoughts most traumatized individuals carry around inside. However, Mike was able to bring those thoughts into our sessions. He told me of his fear that a burglar was going to enter his home at night to rob and kill him. He spent late nights opening every closet, bedroom, and bathroom door and looking under his furniture and beds fearing someone was hiding there. These feelings and thoughts made sense as metaphors for what had happened in Mike's childhood. His father would, in a sense, break into his bedroom at

DOI: 10.4324/9781003215745-8

night and beat him to the point that Mike feared he would be murdered. Mike rationally knew that no one was going to break into his home, but when activated, the intensity of his childhood abuse memories could not be rationalized in the here and now. Thus, Mike did what he could to reassure his traumatized self-states that he was safe.

The breaking down of long-held defenses against remembering or feeling the intensity of his trauma was occurring because our therapeutic relationship had made it safe for Mike to remember and feel his abusive childhood. He was experiencing more of a breakthrough than a full breakdown (Bollas, 2013). Nonetheless, for Mike the feelings were insufferable.

Confronting his parents was not going well because they denied that any abuse had occurred. His anger toward them was often transferred to me. I was also making occasional mistakes that made his projections and transference toward me much more inevitable and intense. At times, Mike was upset that the work was not progressing fast enough. That was understandable, given that he was in the throes of insufferable trauma memories. However, Mike was resilient and determined, and he was able to make use of his anger in the service of healing. He channeled it into his work on his traumas and his commitment to reclaiming and transforming his stolen body.

There were times when Mike needed additional contact with me between sessions. During periods of intense fear and panic, we had almost daily emails, calls, or texts. Often I awoke to emails or texts sent in the middle of the night by an intoxicated Mike. The messages were usually that the feelings he was having were intolerable and that I was not doing my job, that I was not helping him fast enough, that I had assured him all this was going to get better and it was not. Mike's late-night texts were always from his home and were another way of bringing me into his trauma terrors. He was engaging me, even though I was not physically available, knowing I would hear him and his terror when I awoke the next morning. His angry messages, while not what I prefer to wake up to, indicated that Mike was feeling strong enough trust in me and our work that he could express his anger at me without fear of retaliation.

For my part, I worked on not becoming too defensive or expressing my own feelings of despair and fears that Mike was never going to get better, even though on most days I was sure he would. Mike was working too hard not to change and improve. And over time he did feel improvement and began to feel more in control of his trauma memories. After 4 years of treatment, Mike could distinguish his "there-and-then trauma" from his "here-and-now life," including trusting that people did not want to beat him up or murder him. He could also go to bed at night without having to assure himself that no one was hiding and waiting to rob and murder him. These were significant achievements that I seemed to appreciate more than Mike did. Despite the changes, there were still times when his embodied trauma memories haunted him in the present, and he had larger goals than a decent night's sleep. He wanted to transform his emotions and body sensations to the point where his past traumas ceased to haunt him in the present.

Mike knew I worked directly with the body with some patients and had asked me questions about it throughout his work. In year 4, he began reading about embodied trauma and bodywork on the Internet and in books and articles on trauma and the body that I suggested. At this point in our work, there was only limited physical contact between us in the form of an occasional meaningful hug at the end of a session, a form of completion touch. Mike also began receiving occasional massages that we would then process in our sessions.

Unbeknownst to me, Mike had been preparing himself for beginning embodied therapy. He initiated the change in a session in which he not only invited but rather demanded a decision from me to go all-in with the embodied work. I chose to accept his invitation, and we began that work together.

The Beginning of Embodied Therapy

That evening Mike arrived for his session and without talking laid on my couch. This was something he had never done before. The next 50 minutes were an almost surreal experience. Mike's body narrated, or I should say illustrated, his childhood beatings. At times his body looked like he was having some type of seizure because he trembled and convulsed. I was certain I was witnessing what his body looked like during the beatings by his father. I do not think an acclaimed film director could have choreographed the movements with more precision. That was because Mike was not acting. He was completely surrendering to the embodied memories of his abuse and allowing his body to involuntarily release embodied trauma memories, movements, and sensations.

In many ways, Mike's work paralleled my own embodied work from years earlier relative to my asthma attacks (discussed in Chapter 3). My own experience of my body twitching on the massage table helped me to understand this type of work and not become anxious about what I was witnessing. Several times during the session I thought about whether to speak or to move over to the couch and touch Mike. However, I decided to be a silent but intense witness and participant. I observed Mike's body and tried to link each movement to the specific abuse scenes he had described to me. I thought about how a body twitch or movement looked like a child being beaten while he laid in bed. I also noticed and thought about how other body movements and positions seemed to illustrate a child lying all alone in his bed after a severe beating attempting to self-sooth. It was heartbreaking.

As the session neared its end, I spoke first as Mike laid on the couch exhausted and resting with his eyes closed. He opened his eyes to look at me. I gently told him how heartbreaking and moving what I had just witnessed had been. I said that during the session I wanted to come over and put my hand on his shoulder. He said, "I wish you had." I told him that because we had never discussed using touch in a session, I did not think it would be wise to suddenly do that. I did not have his permission to touch him and had been unsure how his traumatized self-states would have received it. I added that I suspected there would be more opportunities for touch because I thought that would not be our last session like this one. Mike responded with a slight smile and an affirming nod of his head.

Our next session began the same way. Mike laid on the couch, and this time I moved my chair next to him and asked if I could place my hand on his shoulder. He nodded and smiled. This began a phase of work that occurred once a week and lasted over 6 months. Trembling and tics in parts of his body (e.g., shoulder, legs) were met with my gentle or firmer touch depending on what seemed needed: softer for comfort, firmer for containment when he trembled. We began to create a structured routine that offered Mike predictability around touch and through which incremental additions to the embodied work could safely be incorporated and processed.

In the early stages of this work, the session routine began with Mike laying face up on the couch, me sitting in a chair facing him, and Mike offering his right hand to hold with my right hand. We would spend 5–10 minutes in that position as Mike updated me on his week. This included any emotions or body sensations he thought I needed to know about and any new memories he had relative to his childhood traumas. When Mike had enough processing, he would roll over on his side facing me, close his eyes, and begin to move into his own intrapsychic space. He would spend some time grounding himself in the safe space between us before moving into intense embodied trauma memories. The shift into these memories was signaled by his body beginning to tremble. Mike would then either remain on his side facing me or roll over onto his stomach. I would move from the chair and onto my knees next to the couch and place one arm around his back and the other resting on his shoulder in what had become a consistent pattern of my using containing–informing touch. This expanded to include times when I would move one of my hands to a specific part of Mike's body that was twitching. When the trembling intensified, I would attempt to create a form of full body containment by placing one hand on his shoulder and the other on his foot and my chest touching his back. This too became part of the predictable routine.

For a period of time in this routine, a verbal addition occurred that was pivotal to the working through of Mike's childhood assaults and terrors from his father. Mike would turn his head toward mine, and I would back up enough to give him space as we made eye contact. In these moments, I could see the terror in Mike's eyes. I believe he could see the empathy in mine. Mike would look straight at me and ask me the same three questions every time:

MIKE: "You're not going to hurt me?"
ED: A firm and empathic "No."

MIKE: "You're not going to kill me?"
ED: Another firm and empathic "No."
MIKE: "You don't hate me?"
ED: A third firm and empathic "No."

Satisfied, and relieved, Mike would smile, lay back on the couch, close his eyes, and we would resume where we left off.

In the fourth week of this verbal exchange, following my own self-processing between sessions, I added one more line to my final response. In our next session, the exchanges were as follows:

MIKE: "You're not going to hurt me?"
ED: A firm empathic "No."
MIKE: "You're not going to kill me?"
ED: Another firm empathic "No."
MIKE: "You don't hate me?"
ED: A third firm and empathic "No."

This was followed by, "I don't hate you; I love you." I said this because the words rang true. My words were met with the reply, "I love you too" and a firm embrace followed. Then, it was back into the routine of the work.

When Mike's embodied trauma flashbacks began to extinguish and he laid on the couch exhausted, my touch gradually began to include completion touch. I would hold his head in my left hand with my right hand around his back. Mike also made use of my embrace as a form of containing–informing touch that enabled him to stay within his own experience and notice what was going on inside his body. I worked on staying attuned to him while also internally and privately processing my own reactions to the work.

Embodied Therapy to Address Mike's Anger and Power

When the work moved from the regressive into the progressive phase, Mike's embodied therapy shifted to addressing his anger and rage toward his parents. I was consulting with a colleague almost weekly to explore possible ways for Mike to address his anger using embodied processes. From these consultations, I decided to begin using more traditional forms of bodywork exercises that fell within the category of somatic mastery and modulation and the hard techniques mentioned in Chapter 2 that Smith (1985) described as more forceful in design in order to address and release blocked energy and emotions.

I had experienced these exercises in the neo-Reichian workshops I attended early in my own bodywork. The emphasis was on helping the participant experience their anger, power, and embodied agency. One form of this work involved a participant pushing against a group leader, making eye contact, and working with the emotions that surfaced. After considering various options, I decided that, given Mike's issues, work around him pushing and using his own strength against my body might work best. This form of body-to-body work could provide him with opportunities to experience his healthy anger and aggression. In many of our previous talk sessions, we had discussed his fear that any expression of his anger would either be met with fierce if not lethal retaliation based on the abuse he experienced from his parents or that his anger would be harmful to someone else.

The work began with my explaining how we would structure the session, beginning in a kneeling position facing each other. We would hold out our hands and push against each other. We were close enough that our elbows were bent, and each of us would have to push to extend them. The idea was to experience pushing against one another in a back and forth manner to help Mike feel both his own and my strength in safe ways. We would finish the session by processing as necessary.

Generally, someone new to this type of exercise tends to begin with apprehension and hesitation, which was true of Mike. The exercise takes some getting used to, including trusting that it is permissible and therapeutic to be physically assertive and aggressive with your therapist. Mike held out his hands and I matched his with my own and waited. We sat there, hands pressed together and looking at one another. After a while, Mike began to push against my hands, and I matched his pressure. Initially his pushing was timid because he was becoming acclimated to the exercise, but as is usually the case, as Mike got used to the experience, he became more aggressive. His pushing became even stronger, and I had to work to maintain my equilibrium. Inevitably, there are times when the patient's pushing is stronger than the therapist's such that the latter's hand and arms are pushed back toward their chest as the patient's hands extend to an almost locked position.

Another common occurrence in this exercise is that the patient feels both confidence and uncertainty in their newfound agency. Generally, uncertainty wins out over confidence in the early sessions. Mike suddenly collapsed his arms to his side, breaking his engagement with me and dejectedly saying, "I can't do this." I remembered saying the same thing in my own work, which helped to inform my response. Taking a slight risk, I responded with, "But you just did it." As I had anticipated, Mike heard my comment as encouraging, and we both appreciated the moment of levity. He chuckled, "I know, but I couldn't keep doing it." I said that getting used to the emotions and body sensations that surfaced as well as his own strength and power was part of the work. He needed to trust that his anger and power would not hurt me—or mine him—and that over time it would get easier to stay with his anger and power.

It did not take many more sessions for Mike to begin enjoying his newfound ability to express his anger and power. In fact, it was all I could do to hold my position without being pushed backward. I began to use the office wall against my back for more support. From that position, Mike was able to push as hard as he wanted because I was anchored against the wall.

Mike's pressure was intense but also controlled, and he continued to make eye contact with me so that his aggression and anger were in full view. Continuing to have one's eyes open in this work is important because it makes it less likely that the patient will dissociate. They can feel and think about their past trauma while being firmly grounded in the here and now and looking at their trusted therapist. An example of this occurred when Mike sometimes said in a raised voice, "I hate you!" There was an implicit understanding that he was thinking about his father as he looked me straight in the eyes. One day after yelling "I hate you!" he added, "I want to kill you!" and his push against my hands intensified. He then broke out of the work for a moment to remind me of something I already knew. He said, "I really don't want to kill you." I replied, "I know you don't want to kill me. I know you don't want to kill anybody. But these are the feelings you had growing up, and I know they are not about me." I smiled and ended with, 'And I love you too.' These exchanges gave Mike permission and confidence to move deeper into his embodied power with less fear and anxiety. He smiled at me and then moved back into an even more intense level of pushing.

In one session, the intensity of our mutual pressure seemed to evoke a spontaneous sense in both of us to move off of our knees and into a standing position where we could make use of our legs. This then became part of the predictable routine. Things progressed to a moment in one session when Mike stopped pushing, put his arms by his side, looked at me, and said, "Would it be possible for you to put your hands around my neck?" I quickly processed in my own mind the possible implications of this move. I decided in Mike's case it would be a safe and informed action given how the work was progressing. I also knew that I would take this work slowly with limited pressure on his neck. I placed my hands around his neck as gently as I could, and he put his hands around my neck. Whenever I do any type of "synchronized work" with a patient, I try to match their movement and their intensity rather than getting ahead of them. So, when Mike's hands were loose around my neck, my hands were loose around his. When he began to apply more pressure, I matched his pressure. During one session, my matching of his firm pressure became too intense for Mike and an embodied flashback of him being strangled was activated. He asked that we stop doing the exercise, which we did. We then sat on the couch and processed the experience. He told me how my hands had felt like his father's and how he was disappointed that we had to discontinue the exercise. I said I understood, apologized for maybe moving too quickly, and assured him that I would get it right the next time.

The next session followed the same predictable pattern of starting on our knees and then shifting to standing up and pushing back and forth until Mike signaled he wanted to focus on work within the neck area. This time we both were more informed and worked at a slower pace. At one point Mike asked if I could remove my hands from his neck and have his remain on mine. For a brief moment I thought about it. I remembered reading of a case (Landy,

2008) where Wilhelm Reich was working with a female patient with a constricted throat and shallow breathing that he theorized was due to her "impulse to choke her mother" (p. 42) who had treated her abusively. Reich had agreed to the patient's request to act out her fantasy of choking him. Landy stated that Reich's patient "acted out her rage cautiously, then let up breathing fully" (p. 42). I had this case in mind as I thought about Mike's request. I was not concerned that Mike would hurt me, but I was quickly processing my concern that Mike might feel that his pressure around my neck would fall into the same category as his father's abuse of him. I decided that if any issues of confusion around that arose we would be able to process them. I then nodded and placed my hands at my side.

For the next several minutes I observed Mike make use of me and my neck to experiment with various forms of pressure and hand positions as we continued to engage in constant eye contact. I observed the multiple reactions he seemed to be having and his calmness and curiosity about what he was doing. This was a slow and detailed process. The most intense moment came when Mike used just enough sustained pressure that I felt my neck being squeezed, though not in a way that created difficulty breathing or created fear in me. I could see in his facial expression a hint of what I would describe as sadistic enjoyment. I thought that this must have been what his father had looked like and that perhaps Mike was trying out what it felt like to have a person in a chokehold the way he described his father's choking him. At no time did Mike forget who he was touching and at no time did I ever feel in danger. Rather, I was moved at Mike's curiosity and his attempts to learn more about his abuse.

When we processed that work, Mike spoke about feeling both power and concern that he might have been hurting me. I assured him that he had not and that the exercise had been helpful in my understanding his trauma in greater detail. I felt like Mike had taken me into that abuse scene from his childhood. I added that the exercise was another way he was learning that he could feel intense anger and at the same time remain in control of his behavior. He was proving to himself he could be angry without hurting others the way his father had hurt him.

Transitional and Progressive Work with Contact Comfort Touching

Following Mike's work around his father's abuse, the therapy shifted to focusing on ways his mother inflicted bodily pain on Mike. He was already processing in talk therapy his anger at his mother for having stood by while his dad beat him, sometimes even encouraging the abuse. Mike was beginning to describe to me many of the ways his mother had also inflicted physical abuse on him. He described how she would use a hard object, such as a yardstick, to hit various parts of his body, including the backs of his ankles, his feet and arms, and buttocks. Almost as bad for Mike was the absence of comforting touch from her, made even worse by his mother's insistence that he massage her body for long periods without any comfort touch from her. Comforting touch was something he desperately wanted and needed from her. It would have provided a different experience of touch that contrasted the abuse.

At my suggestion, Mike began receiving massage from a female massage therapist as a way to work on becoming more comfortable with comforting touch. However, he found the massages did not provide the type of experience he thought would be helpful. He thought part of the issue was his discomfort about focusing on his childhood trauma with a massage therapist he did not know very well. Although the connection with the massage therapist could have deepened over time, Mike was not enthused about having to start over and retell his trauma history with someone new, especially when my touch had been helping him. He felt that continuing embodied work with me would be easier and more effective for him. He asked if I would be willing to engage in the forms of more gentle touch he was looking to explore. I was agreeable, and this began a period of work designed to provide Mike with new forms of contact comfort touch that would also function as containing–informing touch. This work was more progressive as the touch also provided Mike with opportunities to feel and absorb forms of touch that were not provided by his parents and that contrasted with their abuse and his suspicion of physical contact. The following is an example of one aspect of that work.

In the beginning of the work with lighter and comforting forms of touch, Mike would remove his socks and ask if I would rub his feet as a way of relaxing into a calmer state. Sometimes we would process his week during this touch, at other times Mike would just relax into his own private resting space. If I attempted to touch his calf, Mike became somewhat anxious, and although he wanted to tolerate the disruption, in the early stages he usually could not and would have to process the disruption with me. It took weeks for us to develop a predictable routine regarding how he wanted his feet, calves, legs, hands, and arms touched.

Part of the difficulty of this work was that the soft, gentle types of touch Mike requested were challenging for me to provide as he lay on the couch because it took so much concentration and coordination. Mike lying on the couch and me on a chair or standing beside the couch created awkward positions that were difficult for me to sustain for long periods. After a month I decided I could more effectively create the type of embodied resting space Mike wanted by using my massage table. I spoke with him about moving to the massage table and he was agreeable. This work was never referred to as traditional massage. There were no scented candles or music creating a specific atmosphere. Mike did not remove his clothing and did not lie under a sheet with a heated table, and I did not perform a standard massage. However, there was a bottom sheet covering the table and a pillow on which Mike rested his head. He usually took his socks off and wore shorts and a loose t-shirt for easier access to his arms, hands, back, legs, and feet.

With Mike on the massage table, I was able to provide the light touch he was requesting for the full 50-minute session. This touch seemed to evoke childhood states in Mike that he would relax into privately and in silence for most of the session. An important part of each session was Mike needing to guide me as to when and where to move to another part of his body. In each session he wanted different sections of his body addressed depending on what trauma memories were more pronounced. In this way, Mike was also gaining confidence that his requests would be taken seriously without me laughing or shaming him, something that had occurred so often in his childhood.

Such work in body analysis with trauma can sometimes be complicated. Some days my touch felt exclusively comforting, thus allowing Mike to sink deeply into his own internal experience and feel what embodied care was supposed to have felt like in childhood. On other days this private and safe resting place would be intruded on by an abuse memory. Sometimes that memory came with Mike to a session, at other times it occurred while he was on the table. Even a subtle way I touched him could activate an embodied trauma memory. For instance, my light touch of his calf early in the work evoked somatic memories of his calves being smacked by his mother.

The work shifted to focusing on Mike becoming comfortable with a combination of soft and firm touch. The lighter, softer forms of touch felt the best to him, but given that his mom would use soft touch prior to initiating abuse, Mike often became suspicious of it. He suggested that I begin to occasionally contrast the soft touch with firm but not hard touch as a way to perhaps help break his fear of comforting touch turning abusive. I never seemed to be able to get it exactly right because I never knew when to shift from soft to firm touch. However, Mike was never angry at me during those misattunements and understood them as part of the work. We verbally processed those moments either when they occurred or at the end of the session. Mike helped me to learn more about the specific nuances of how his body remembered the before, during, and after of his abuse.

Over time, Mike's body continued to become more comfortable with my touch and not flinch if it was sometimes too firm. He would lie on the massage table for the full session without either of us saying a word other than Mike informing me where to focus my touch. In that way, we both felt the work was providing him with a new experience of being soothed by another's touch. Mike began to notice a reduction in his chronic anxiety to the point where his anxiety was becoming more acute and situational. The weekly massage table work also became a type of independent study whereby Mike would privately self-analyze the impact my touch was having on various self-states and trauma memories. Sometimes, he shared an insight but most of the time his thoughts remained private. The absence of more processing in this phase was comfortable for me because we had done so much processing to get to that space. In addition, during the course of a session, I felt deeply attuned to Mike and his body and could feel the mutual attunement between us. The sessions continued this way for over 2 years, during which Mike's ability to ask for comforting touch from his wife expanded as well.

The work with Mike described in this chapter shows how the progressive phase can provide patients with a new experience of touch that can be internalized and then used in other relationships. Mike's embodied therapy could have been considered successful even if the work had only helped him deal with his embodied trauma flashbacks. However, the two of us were able to take the work a step further by moving into a more progressive phase in which he could now rest and experience pleasurable touch without fear or suspicion. That provided him with a more expansive transformation of his stolen body. Although more work was needed, the embodied therapy that began 4 years into Mike's nontouch psychoanalytic psychotherapy became anchored in progressive forms of treatment. The combination of psychoanalytic psychotherapy and embodied therapy was instrumental in helping him transform his experience of his physical abuse and neglect within both his mind and his body.

Reference

Bollas, C. (2013). *Catch them before they fall: The psychoanalysis of breakdown*. Routledge. doi:10.4324/9780203069547.

Landy, R. J. (2008) *The couch and the stage: Integrating words and action in psychotherapy*. Jason Aronson.

Smith, E. W. L. (1985). *The body in psychotherapy*. McFarland & Co.

Chapter 8

Jodie
Childhood Trauma

The next three chapters provide details about the 8-year combined psycho-analysis and body analysis I did with a patient. It began as talk therapy and progressed to include all five categories of touch and three phases of embodied treatment as outlined in Chapter 2.

Jodie was in her late thirties and seeking treatment for what she described in her email as "issues from childhood." In the first 6 months of our work together, she told me little about her traumas other than that her grandfather had been sexually abusive during her visits to her grandparent's house when she was a child. Slowly I learned these were weekly visits. Jodie's grandmother was an accomplice in the sexual abuse, and Jodie appeared to have been singled out while the other grandchildren played in other rooms or went shopping with their grandmother. Jodie also suspected her grandfather had abused his own daughters, Jodie's aunts, when they were young. Those horrific weekly visits occurred when Jodie was 4 to 7 years old and often included overnight stays. Finally, when Jodie was 7, her grandparents moved out of state and the visits stopped.

For many months in our work, those were all the verbal details I heard about the abuse. In addition, there were limited indications that Jodie had any connection with that younger part of herself. In fact, until our work, Jodie had never really thought about her childhood. However, although she could not recognize her younger self states, I began to see, think about, and experience them. Although Jodie talked little about the details of those awful days and nights with her grandparents, her body showed and told me about the experience in multiple ways: She made almost no eye contact, an almost inaudible and quivering voice, stiff if not frozen body posture, quivering shoulders, and a nervous stomach connected to irritable bowel syndrome (IBS) that Jodie had lived with since childhood. Her arrivals and departures from sessions were without eye contact, and if she did look in my direction, her head was generally bent toward the ground. It seemed I was in the presence of the body presentation of her as a 4-to-7-year-old traumatized child.

Jodie's way of being in sessions was remarkably different from the adult woman outside my office (whom I actually felt intimidated by) and the one

DOI: 10.4324/9781003215745-9

she presented to the world outside. She was bright, well educated, and worked hard at everything she committed to doing. Her educational background was in child psychology, and she spent her career focusing on protecting and helping children. Jodie was also a wonderful mother to her own three children. She had been a competitive athlete in high school and college and continued to push her body athletically. I began to learn that Jodie related to her body more like a machine that she expected to perform at high levels with limited rest or self-care.

A Body Speaks

Although Jodie spent most of her session time in verbal silence, I felt a connection developing between us. During the often long silences, I had ample time to observe and think. The silence in that early work was almost never pleasant. There was a traumatic quality to it, as if the atmosphere of her grandparent's home was filling what should have been the sacred and safe space of my office. I often thought about what being in her grandparent's house must have felt like to her, including the torturous anticipation on Fridays of having to go there over the weekend.

In sessions, I experienced Jodie as cut off from me and alone. She seemed to be predominately regressed within her childhood trauma and self-states, even though she could not yet recognize that this was happening. I saw my job was to remain attuned to and observant with her, to notice when she seemed more available to engaging with me and when the session required my empathic attunement from a distance. I also paid attention to my own internal experiences and thought about how I could use them to inform our work. When Jodie shifted into a more here-and-now adult self-state, she would spend the session talking about what was going on in her current life, including her job, children, and family events. Sometimes she talked about how she was beginning to make connections between her childhood trauma and the impact it was still having on her. At those times, I could engage with her in forms of psychoeducation around trauma, including introducing the idea of self-states using transactional analytic and psychoanalytic theories.

When Jodie moved into longer periods of silence, I witnessed and felt her traumatized self-states within her body movements, facial expressions, voice, and silence. I learned that there were two types of silence for her. One was here-and-now adult contemplative silence. The other was more of an internal psychic withdrawal, reminiscent of her coming home from her grandparents, going to her room, and curling up in bed for hours. In these moments, Jodie showed me the pain, sadness, and shock in the aftermath of an abusive weekend. Through that regressive work, I learned more about Jodie's trauma through her silence and her body than through a detailed narrative. I also became more in tune with these two types of silence, which helped me adjust my presence and engagement with Jodie to match the self-state she was experiencing.

Slowly and quietly, without eye contact and holding on to her scarf or her hands, Jodie talked about her grandfather lying next to her and masturbating while touching her and calling her "a dirty little girl." She also remembered her grandmother telling her that she was a "dirty little girl" and accusing Jodie of wanting her grandfather "to do those things to her." The words "dirty little girl" had been taken literally by her. She said to this day, she had difficulty feeling her body was not dirty when someone touched her. She talked about her grandfather's anger when she cried or would not comply with his demands and how she learned to lay there mostly motionless and silent. I thought about how this might be linked to the freeze state I saw in her so often.

Jodie told me about the ways she tried to avoid having to be alone with her grandfather, including trying to stay close to her cousins. She also avoided eye contact, believing somehow the abuse was her fault and maybe had to do with eye contact. I internally speculated that perhaps this was why she was not making eye contact with me. I also learned her grandfather would abuse her in either the bathroom or the bedroom. Some days when she arrived, he would give her a children's sedative cold medicine to make her drowsy. Later I learned of one time another grandchild inquired, "Why are you giving her that? She's not even sick." She told of an aunt who suggested to Jodie, "Pretend you are sleeping," something Jodie now suspected the aunt had tried unsuccessfully in her own childhood.

In an almost inaudible whisper, Jodie told me that each weekend, after her grandfather's abuse, she would go out in the family room and wrap herself up in a blanket on the couch. While the other kids played, Jodie laid on the couch almost motionless until the parents came to pick up their children. To make things even worse, Jodie's parents would make sure she gave grandpa a hug and kiss before they left, and they became angry with her when she resisted.

The theme of Jodie's parents not seeing and observing her continued to deepen in the therapy. She told me of times she "hinted" at the abuse in conversations with her mother.

MOTHER: Why don't you like going over there?
JODIE: Grandpa touches me, he tickles me too hard, he does things to me.
MOTHER: Oh! Don't say such bad things about you grandfather. That's not nice.

Later in treatment, Jodie remembered at age 7 telling her mother directly what was happening. Her mother became angry, called her a liar, and walked away. Jodie said that was the moment she decided never again to tell anyone because being disbelieved was too devastating. In fact, I was the first person after that to hear about her traumas. However, I was seeing and feeling them more than hearing about them. What Jodie and I did not know at the time was that Jodie's decision to avoid the devastation of another person not believing her was part of our therapeutic relationship. Despite our good therapeutic fit, Jodie's fear of me not believing her was powerful. Years later, as we processed this period in her therapy, we concluded that the fear of me not believing her was too intense for her to push through. In what I believe was a brilliant and unconscious decision on her part, Jodie showed me the trauma using her body and embodied communication.

Jodie was able to create the type of therapy she needed in order to trust me with her traumatized self. She needed me to feel both her emotions and embodied trauma memories slowly, over time, to see that each specific movement and memory was known and believed by me, before she could move to another part of her abuse history. She also needed me to develop a relationship with her childhood traumatized body and self-state.

When she shifted into an embodied trauma memory, I became a witness to her abuse. I would sit in the silence and watch Jodie slipping away from me and the present and back into her strong defense of internal self-isolation. In these moments, I made mistakes around attempts at encouraging her to talk and make eye contact. I was trying to have her engage with me with limited success. It took many weeks before I began to understand what would eventually become a common theme in our work. I needed to go back into the regressive experience with her and meet her in those childhood traumas rather than continuing to try to pull her into the present, to get to know her and her traumas within her embodied sensations and silence.

I became more attuned to Jodie's suffering, which she had endured in silence most of her life, as I was gradually invited into her history of suffering. As our relationship deepened, I noticed that I wanted to move closer to her, maybe even touch and comfort her. That is not an unusual response for a therapist working with childhood trauma, especially when there is a strong connection between the therapist and patient. However, in Jodie's case, I experienced this pull toward empathic touch and contact comfort more intensely than usual. I believe this was because she was showing me her trauma more than telling me. Because her primary way of telling me about her trauma was through her body, she needed someone intently attuned to her physically.

As I said, as Jodie's embodied trauma memories continued to surface, I was motivated to provide comfort and containment for her. Sitting across from her felt like repeating her childhood experience, when she spent her time alone in the aftermath of the abuse. Perhaps most noticeable to me were Jodie's hands, which were almost the only active part of her body. Often they were engaged with one another, for example, in hand wringing. She often wore a long scarf around her neck and shoulders. Often she would grab each end of the scarf as if she were holding on for protection, support, and what I thought might be a long-standing desire for connection and comfort.

Jodie and I first began working in the terrain of the body by processing the impact sexual abuse can have on a child's thoughts about touch and their relationship with their own body. She had been curious about my work in body psychotherapy, and we sometimes discussed if and how that kind of work might be appropriate for her. Although curious about embodied therapy, Jodie was apprehensive about engaging in physical contact. Her primary fears were not that I would abuse her but that I would think she was doing something wrong or that I would feel her body was "dirty" as her grandparents had. For months we continued discussions around embodied therapy to help both of us to understand how to avoid any form of physical touch that could have been misunderstood by or harmful to her.

One day I decided to talk about using touch in her therapy, about how sad and lonely she looked and felt to me. I speculated that might have been how she felt as a little girl, and she agreed. I also described my thoughts about moving my chair next to hers and possibly holding her hand rather than her having to find comfort in her scarf. I knew my comment risked shaming Jodie over her use of the scarf, but my comment carried the empathic feelings I was having for her. Her slight nod confirmed that my comment resonated with her experience, so I added that I thought, despite perhaps wanting to hold my hand, she might be feeling scared and anxious. Another slight nod from Jodie. I ended the discussion with the possibility of embodied work by saying that we would not move into any forms of touch until and if she was ready and that it was on her terms. She again nodded and let out what seemed to be a sigh of relief.

After consultation with some colleagues and several more discussions with Jodie about the possibility of touch, we made the decision to include some form of embodied work into the therapy. We started by sitting next to one another in my office chairs. Even after I moved my chair next to hers, there were many sessions before we incorporated touch into her work. From the time I moved my chair until the time she reached for my hand, there was almost another month of nontouch sessions. During that time, we had two sessions a week and continued to talk and process as best we could, but the verbal work was clearly limited. Jodie remained predominately silent and focused on her own thoughts and body sensations. She did, however, continue to be more curious about her embodied trauma memories and occasionally could tell me what she was noticing in her body, including wanting to hold my hand. She could also speak to how anxious she became when she thought about that. Sometimes she would look at my hand resting on the armrest of my chair. Her apprehension and inability to reach for my hand was agonizing for both of us. She told me about how fearful she was that I would "blame her" for something, that I might misinterpret her touch as sexual or even feel she was the "dirty little girl" her grandparents had made her out to be.

Why I Did Not Reach for Her Hand

There were several reasons why I did not reach over and hold Jodie's hand. First, my training in bodywork had always emphasized the patient's own embodied agency. Such work was designed to help the person to feel and experience their own body as an active participant rather than in more passive ways. The work with Jodie slightly changed my position on that, especially when working with early childhood traumas. I no longer hold such a strong position that the work is primarily about the patient claiming their own body agency and vitality. Rather, I believe the patient's ability to take in safe and empathic touch from their therapist is equally important in helping the person to reclaim their stolen body and transform embodied trauma. I also believe when working with embodied trauma, the therapist needs to talk about their own informed thoughts relative to touch and sometimes take the lead in initiating touch depending on the trauma and the patient. The patient maintains an active role in both the contract around touch and the processing of any touch.

In Jodie's case, I could see and she reported that she was learning more about her trauma by internally reflecting on both her desire and her anxiety over possibly holding my hand. She did not feel like I was withholding touch from her by my not reaching for her hand. In fact, she said that while me reaching for her hand would make things easier, she felt that it was important for her to initiate the first hand holding.

Our First Embodied Contact

When the day came that Jodie reached for my hand, there were only 5 minutes left in the session. There had been a lengthy period of silence as she stared at my hand. Suddenly, she reached over and took it. To me, Jodie's hand felt more like that of a child rather than a strong adult. It felt small and inert, with limited movement or vitality. Internally, I felt empathic and somewhat parental as I thought about her childhood traumas and how difficult it was trusting me with this private and guarded part of herself. We sat motionless, just noticing our hands in contact. I would say at that moment there was probably nothing comforting about the contact for Jodie. The best that could be said was that it was containing–informing touch or maybe the beginning of what would come to be somatic mastery and modulation. Mostly I sensed what seemed to be a huge relief for Jodie that she had finally connected with my hand.

During the following months, hand holding became a predictable part of Jodie's sessions. We would sit next to one another for approximately 10 minutes in silence. Jodie would fall into an internal experiential space that she used to become reacquainted with her childhood trauma, my office, the therapeutic space, and my presence. That ritual helped her feel safe and ready to then reach for my hand. Slowly, reaching for my hand became easier, even though Jodie still sat in silence for most of each session. However, in a soft voice, she described how she was beginning to feel a closer connection to both me and her childhood self.

Gradually, both of our hands became more active, and we began taking turns initiating various hand movements, although Jodie preferred me to initiate early in that work. We noticed how different hand positions were experienced by her. Sometimes our hands would rest on the chair armrest with my hand on top of hers. At other times her hand would rest on top of mine. Sometimes I would hold her hand in mine, at other times she held mine in hers. Hand in hand seemed to connect to her childhood self-states. Our fingers interlocking felt more like a here-and-now adult sensation to her. Jodie was exploring both of these positions and was finding that if the move into her childhood trauma was too intense, she could shift to interlocking fingers to ground herself in the here and now.

We processed how she experienced the hand holding: "strange," "comforting," "remarkable" were some of the words she used. She was also learning what forms of contact seemed a better fit for her trauma. One of the most important parts of this period was her increased understanding of how uncomfortable, ashamed, and critical she was of her own body and how difficult it was for her to feel comfortable touching and interacting with another person's body.

As the work with hand holding expanded, there was another subtle addition to the routine: the interaction between two thumbs, my right and her left. Spontaneously, one day we put our thumbs together and Jodie began using our thumbs as a safe and uncomplicated way of analyzing her body in relationship to mine by alternating pushing softly and firmly against my thumb. Sometimes, we were both pushing just about as hard as we could. Jodie began to explore pinning my thumb against the armrest of the chair. Often I would then repeat her move with slightly less pressure. I watched her looking at our thumbs, moving hers into different positions and pushing against mine with different pressures. I thought about what each movement might mean for her, and we usually processed all of this at the end of the session. I was surprised how much a slight shift in hand positions could change the experience for Jodie.

There were still long silences and no eye contact from Jodie, even within our hand holding and thumb connections. In our processing, I linked her pushing of my thumb to aggression and speculated that this could be anger toward her grandparents and parents. In retrospect, I think the intense thumb pressure was less about aggression and more about a desire for connection with me. But thinking about aggression, rather than her strong desire for connection, was how I was trained to think about bodywork.

Several weeks into that work, Jodie asked if we could switch sides so she could experience that work with her right hand. The shift in chairs created new explorations and connections because Jodie seemed more comfortable and less inhibited in the second chair. What we had discovered was that the routine of the sessions helped her feel more comfortable adding to and expanding the work with touch as she became more familiar and confident with the work. In the second chair, Jodie's hand was more expressive. There were times her hand felt and acted in more adult ways, such as firmer and stronger holding of my hand. I also continued to experience a difference between interlocking fingers and hands cupped together. In processing she stated that cupped hands felt more comforting, whereas interlocked fingers felt more like an adult-to-adult connection.

During this phase, Jodie was often cold in sessions, which seemed to be part of her fear response because my office was not cold, at least not to me and most other patients. I offered Jodie a blanket, and she decided to use it to keep warm. This led to her beginning each office session by covering herself with the blanket. That seemed connected to her covering herself up and sleeping following her childhood abuse. By using the blanket in session, Jodie felt she was able to re-create and explore her childhood attempts at self-soothing and repair. I suggested she could also use the blanket to help inform our work with touch and that I would not touch any part of her body that was under the blanket. That idea was influenced by the actions of her grandfather, who often molested her underneath the blankets at night when she was sleeping. I did not want to evoke that trauma. The blanket also helped Jodie let me know what parts of her body she wanted to address in a session. She always began covered by the blanket, with only her left hand exposed. Gradually, she then moved the blanket off an arm or shoulder when she was ready for more contact.

Another sense that Jodie began to make use of and that became an important part of the work was smell and scent. Apparently, the blanket had picked up my specific scent. Ironically, over time, to me the blanket had more of Jodie's lotion smell than my own scent. She had a remarkable way of making use of my scent in ways that seemed to seep in and comfort her. She started taking the blanket home between sessions and on weekends to help her stay connected to both me and her child self-states. She would also cover herself up on her couch at home during her early phone sessions. These were the beginnings of Jodie's progressive work, which would lead to her being able to create for herself internal forms of psychic and embodied resting.

Jodie's Head Resting on My Shoulder

For weeks I occasionally noticed Jodie staring somewhat curiously at my shoulder. One day when she was doing that, I asked what she was thinking. After more silence, she talked about having thoughts of resting her head on my shoulder, although she had been afraid to ask to do that. Jodie's apprehensions were primarily around her childhood traumas and her fears she would do something wrong, that I would think she was seducing me or that she was "dirty." My reassurance that her expressing such a concern, and even her request, would be welcomed reduced some of her apprehension and opened up our ability to think about and process what that might be like for her. Over time, and with more discussion, Jodie became confident that resting her head on my shoulder would not be misunderstood by me and could be an important addition to her treatment.

One day in the middle of a session, Jodie asked if she could place her head on my shoulder. That seemed like a natural extension of our hands and arms being in contact. Despite some initial apprehension, Jodie quickly became comfortable with that new addition to her sessions. She would begin the first 10 minutes of each session sitting silently under the blanket in her own safe resting space before reaching for my hand. After taking time to absorb the touch and smells of this safe and reparative space, Jodie would then move to rest her head on my shoulder. When she was ready, we would then switch chairs and complete the same established routine from the other side. This helped create the type of sacred space Jodie needed to engage in the forms of embodied connections necessary for transforming her childhood traumas.

During this phase, Jodie started to find her "trauma voice." She began to provide more details about her abuse. This included where and how her grandfather touched her, more of the ways he talked to her, and more detail around grandma's involvement in helping him be alone with Jodie. As she spoke, I experienced her body feeling like it was in the child self-state. She would be covered with the blanket with only her hand outside in order to hold my hand. I experienced her as being in a terrorized frozen state reminiscent of her childhood. There would then be a gradual progression from being frozen to being, as she said, "completely relaxed" by the end of the session. Jodie said she felt her body was predominantly in an embodied childhood state but that she was now able to remain present and curious within a strong observing adult self. This was significant because she was not becoming overwhelmed with trauma. I believe the slow, careful pacing of the work was crucial to this process.

In some sessions, Jodie remembered more details of her abuse. Following a new disclosure, she would become verbally silent and turn inward to stay within her emotions and thoughts about the new memory. My job was to remain present to her through the physical connections we had established so she could feel my presence without having to look at or engage verbally with me, thereby interrupting her important intrapsychic processing.

Jodie was speaking more, but her volume did not increase. In an almost inaudible whisper, she would tell me what she was remembering, and I would try to follow. However, the combination of her almost inaudible whisper and my early-onset hearing loss at times made it impossible for me to hear what she was saying. I found myself straining to hear her important words and disclosures, and I spontaneously moved closer to her in order to hear. In my straining to hear, my head moved closer to her face. In this position, I could also see and feel her shoulder twitches and hear her stomach growling. One day I noticed—and I was not sure how long this had been occurring—that my forehead was resting against hers and we were almost cheek to cheek. My initial reaction was concern because I thought that spontaneous shift in my position might be too intrusive. But I noticed Jodie did not seem that concerned about where my head was. She was engaged in her own intrapsychic experience. I believe her comfort with this spontaneous shift was due, in part, to the predictable pattern and routine of touch that had been established in our work. At the end of the session, we processed how my head was touching hers, and Jodie affirmed she was comfortable with that closeness and that the physical contact helped her contain her anxiety and body sensations as she thought more deeply about her trauma.

For Jodie, there were still apprehensions, fears, feelings that her body was disgusting, that she was doing something wrong and that I was going to see her as the "dirty little girl." However, there were also feelings of being known, cared for, and loved. Slowly, we were transforming, reconfiguring, and healing her abuse from her grandparents. Jodie was gradually reclaiming both her child self, which had been split off, and her body. She was also becoming unfrozen in the way she held her body in session and was beginning to forge a connection with her own child self-states. This included the new experience of how being in physical contact could feel safe and good rather than abusive or dirty.

As the embodied therapy expanded, Jodie was also developing an increased capacity to not only experience my touch as safe but to feel safer in touching me as well. She was beginning to move from holding my hand to experimenting with touching my arm in various ways. This always resulted in an initial nervous shoulder twitch as she was still apprehensive about whether her touch would feel dirty or suspicious to me. Jodie also feared her initiation of touch would be experienced as sexual and shift me (i.e., a man) into then touching her sexually, with her being blamed for "seducing him." In our work and processing, she began to trust her own ability to touch me without exciting me and that all touch did not lead to her being sexualized.

Whenever a new memory surfaced, Jodie's stomach began churning, and her right shoulder twitched. I continued to learn details about specific self-states and her trauma from my body contact and body proximity with her. Movements such as a shoulder twitch could indicate the severity of a trauma memory based on the intensity of the movement. Locked fingers signaled a more adult-to-adult connection, whereas cupped hands indicated a child-to-adult connection. Shallow breathing and growling stomach informed me about how stirred up Jodie was and how active I might need to be in helping her contain her emotions and body sensations. In my own analytic observing space during sessions, I analyzed what forms of touch seemed most effective, what touch might activate an embodied trauma flashback, and what touch was more effective when Jodie was more regressed or more adult. I also internally reflected on what I was noticing about her within my own embodied reactions.

Jodie was finding a newfound peace in being able to sit with me and enjoy being both held by me and holding me as well. She believed that the embodied therapy was essential in allowing her to both speak and feel her traumas without becoming overwhelmed. She said that when feelings of her abuse surfaced, our physical connection helped her feel safe, known, and understood. In this way, the containing–informing touch as well as contact comfort touch allowed her to stay with her trauma memories without becoming flooded and to make comparisons between her there-and-then trauma and the here-and-now experience with me. The work was certainly nonlinear because a present-day event could activate her childhood trauma. This would then be addressed and processed within the session using the predictable pattern of physical contact that was now part of her sessions. It would be only a few months until a new disclosure created both new challenges and new pathways of embodied connection and embodied transformation in her treatment.

Chapter 9

Jodie
Adult Trauma

One day, Jodie's session began with a different kind of silence. With her head on my shoulder, I could sense restlessness and discomfort in her. I was confused, and she did not reply to my question "What's going on?" We had three or four sessions in a row like that where Jodie seemed unable to get comfortable with me, the work, or her body. My own confusion and anxiety increased. I found it difficult to create embodied attunement because nothing felt right. There were moments when I seemed attuned with Jodie, but even those fell short of what I had felt before in our work. I experienced increased twitching in Jodie's shoulder, her head buried into my shoulder with no verbal engagement with me, her irregular breathing and intense stomach noises. I could not locate any sense of Jodie's child self-states or traumas and was having difficulty figuring out how to relate to her.

Then, in one session, after about 20 minutes, Jodie said in a soft whisper—which sadly I did not hear the first time but only when she repeated it—that she had been raped. I later learned the details. When she was 24 and in graduate school, she was working a part-time job. An older man she worked with had drugged her soda during work hours and then violently raped her after the store closed for the evening. She had never told anyone about this assault because it appears she had been in deep shock, confusion, and dissociation for weeks after the attack. Following this disclosure, she collapsed, burying her head even deeper between my shoulder blade and the chair, silent and frozen. There was no bodily evidence of her child self-states, only a broken 24-year-old young woman.

We sat in this painful silence for a long time. Occasionally I would offer a few words of empathy, just to remind her I was still with her, but I primarily just held her in contact comfort. I asked if I could put my hand on her head and she slightly nodded. We sat there together, she in her own trauma, deadness, and shame, me feeling a pull to do more for her and knowing all she could tolerate and needed at the moment was my unintrusive physical presence.

This new disclosure led to Jodie moving inward for the next few months, a defensive solitude that at times I found difficult to tolerate. Her primary way

DOI: 10.4324/9781003215745-10

of dealing with her traumas had been to shut the world out, and now she was shutting me out as well. I wanted to be in this reliving of the trauma memories and emotions with her. I wanted to talk, process, hold her in a completion touch hug at the end of sessions. Jodie was not ready for any embodied therapy about her college trauma and requested only that I remain physically present to her in session and occasionally hold her hand.

A difference between the childhood and college traumas was that the child self-states wanted both to touch and be touched, whereas within the college trauma Jodie wanted to remain physically separate from me. In fact, I would not have even begun to engage in embodied therapy as early as I had if I had known about the rape. Jodie insisted that she did not want to stop the embodied therapy, especially because she was finding the work with her childhood traumas productive and transformative. I was left having to figure out how to work differently with these two different traumas.

Embodied Mistakes

During this phase of the work, I made several mistakes. I was gradually discovering that how or where I touched Jodie depended on which trauma was primary in the session. Touching Jodie's neck and arms was safe and welcomed when working with her childhood abuses. However, when she shifted into the college trauma, touching her arms could activate or intensify her embodied flashbacks. I learned that when Jodie was experiencing the rape, her neck was never a safe or comforting place to touch and would activate an intense embodied flashback of possibly being choked during her assault.

Her right shoulder blade was different in that both trauma states responded well to that physical contact. There were times when Jodie requested I use my hand to push against her shoulder blade. We began to discover that my hand on her shoulder blade only felt safe to Jodie after she first became reacquainted with my body in our routine, that is, after an initial period of silence, followed by hand holding, then her head on my shoulder. Only then could she make use of my hand against her shoulder blade as a form of comfort and containment within her college trauma memories. Eventually, my touching her shoulder blade expanded to include a welcomed and mutual hug or embrace on the chairs near the end of the session.

As described in Chapter 8, Jodie's childhood self-state experiences found our skin-to-skin contact essential to the work. I was becoming more attuned to which trauma was primary in the beginning of a session by the type of shirt Jodie wore. A shirt like a tank top that exposed her arms signaled childhood self-state work. When the college trauma was primary, Jodie wore shirts that covered her shoulders. One day, during a summer heat wave, Jodie wore a long-sleeved winter shirt. That session was steeped in her college trauma. I was careful to wait several sessions until the timing seemed appropriate to ask about her choice of clothing to avoid possibly shaming or making her feel self-conscious. Jodie reported being completely unaware of her clothing choices, but she became curious about the connection between the clothes she wore and the trauma to which they might be connected. In that way, even her clothing was helping to inform our work.

A mistake I made more than once was attempting to move from contact comfort into somatic mastery and modulation too soon. Once again, this was due to my training, which had been critical of contact comfort because it was thought that forms of comfort touch focused too much on emotional corrective experiences and not enough on the patient's embodied agency and vitality. I now understand that often contact comfort is essential, especially in the early stages of trauma work. By first engaging in contact comfort while working in the regressive phase, the patient can then begin to make better use of more advanced forms of touch in the transitional and progressive phases. I was beginning to understand that Jodie would first need forms of comfort touch within the work on her college trauma memories to help her from becoming overwhelmed by them.

Prior to this understanding, and true to my training, I focused on getting Jodie to "feel her own strength" or "engage in her own vitality." One exercise we tried was to have Jodie pushing back on my hands. Another was both of us standing facing each other with Jodie pushing against my chest or arms. These exercises almost always resulted in an embodied flashback that sometimes had her collapsing into the chair and going silent for the rest of the session. Eventually, I began to understand it was way too early in her treatment for such work and that it might never be the treatment of choice for her. I moved away from that type of bodywork with Jodie, realizing that I was trying to mold her treatment into trauma theory and bodywork techniques rather than paying more attention to her specific treatment needs.

Through my peer consultations, I also discovered that my motivations to help Jodie feel her strength were also due, in part, to my own abuse issues. Helping her feel strength and vitality felt safer and less anxiety provoking for me than engaging in soft, nurturing, and comforting touch that I worried could feel suspicious or be misinterpreted and result in my being blamed for having done something wrong. This often led to what I believe is a common mistake around touch: the therapist pulling back from the embodied work out of their own anxiety and fear rather than as a result of a more informed decision.

I will next give an example of where, in session with Jodie, my own anxiety led to a withdrawal and powerful enactment.

An Embodied Mistake Followed by an Analytic Enactment

In one particular session, there had been a solid embodied connection within both Jodie's childhood and college traumas, and they seemed more integrated. As we neared the session's end, I thought perhaps I could reintroduce working on her body memories of possibly being choked during her rape. I moved my hand slightly off of her shoulder so that it was resting between her shoulder and the side of her neck. This was a shift that in past sessions generally resulted in anxiety for her, and so we had stopped attempting it. But because some time had passed, the work on her college trauma was gaining traction, and she was feeling so safe, I thought we might be able to create a new experience of touch around her neck. In retrospect, this could be viewed as both a procedural and a clinical mistake as defined in Chapter 7. Procedurally, Jodie was not ready to engage in this form of touch within her college trauma, and she could not make use of the physical connection. Clinically, my touching near her neck did not match the type of touch Jodie was expecting in that moment.

Both catching Jodie off guard and the actual contact on the side of her neck activated embodied flashbacks of her college assault. Jodie pushed me away, and I could tell from the look on her face that she was confused if not somewhat dissociated as evidenced by a lack of eye contact and the look someone has when just waking up. Being in that type of situation is never good near the end of a session because there is so little time to process what is happening. I believe at a body level Jodie had experienced a trauma reenactment, and we were about to move into an enactment in the processing.

The enactment in that case was the result of my own childhood traumas, in which I was repeatedly accused of nonconsensual sexual touch by my mother. My own childhood feelings of being bad and lecherous were activated, and even though I could sense where my response was coming from, I just could not stop my defensive response of attempting to explain and justify the movement of my hand as wanting to help Jodie feel OK with touch around her neck. That explanation was certainly accurate, but it was irrelevant to Jodie in the moment. I continued with my defensive explanations, invoking the kind of analytic jargon one might revert to when stuck in their own fears and anxiety around touch. Jodie heard my theoretical explanations as though I was blaming her. She had had enough of that in childhood. The session ended with Jodie still feeling confused and angered by my actions. We agreed to continue processing more over the phone the next day.

At the time, I did not fully understand that at this level of work, body analysis, like psychoanalytic psychotherapy, can include intense mistakes of this nature when working with trauma. If I had, I might not have become anxious and defensive. I might have been able to stay with and process Jodie's reactions rather than justifying my mistake.

The next day we processed both the embodied mistake and the resulting enactment. Jodie was more confused and upset about my attempts at explaining my touching her neck than at the actual embodied mistake. We seemed to do a fairly good job of repairing in the phone session, but Jodie felt there was something still not quite right. She thought that my attempts at explaining my motivations following the embodied mistake had been out of character for me. She wanted to process more in our next face-to-face session.

We began that session sitting on the chairs without any touch. I remained silent, which afforded Jodie the opportunity to take her time and tell me what she needed me to understand. She mentioned how devastating the last embodied session had been because she needed me with her. She said I had promised to be with her in this work and that she was leaning on me and trusting me with her traumas. But she felt that I had abandoned her in the last session. She restated that although processing in the phone session had been helpful, something still felt incomplete and missing. At that moment, I had a decision to make. How much should I disclose of my own issues? Jodie was correct that I had made a therapeutic all-in commitment to her and her work. In addition, she sensed I was withholding part of my reaction. Based on my commitment to her, her sensing there was something unfinished, and because I believed my disclosure would be therapeutic, I decided to speak to my issues.

I told her that in the last session, when she moved into a more dissociated space created by my mistake, the confused look on her face and the way she was talking reminded me of how my mother looked when blaming me for her sexual abuse of me. I told Jodie I had become defensive in not wanting to again be falsely accused of sexually abusing someone. I said I knew Jodie was not blaming me of abusing her even though that was what had become activated in me. I added that my fear in saying all this was that she would again feel like I was blaming her, which I was not. I fell silent and held my breath. Jodie was moved by my disclosure. She said no one had ever been that honest with her about any transgression in her childhood abuse. Now I was owning up to a mistake rather than blaming her. She felt my disclosure had been the missing piece, and she was correct that it was. She hugged me and we held the embrace. It was a form of repair and completion touch for both of us but asymmetrically tilted toward her. The trust within our therapeutic relationship deepened, and the work continued.

Working with Two Different Traumas

The next 6 months of treatment were brutal. Jodie was often unsure of what she needed, and I was struggling to understand what forms of embodied work would be helpful. This was because we were working with two different forms of embodied trauma requiring two different forms of embodied therapy.

The childhood traumas had been chronic, continuing for 3 years during her early childhood development. The perpetrators were revered family members and other family members who either did not notice the abuse or looked away. Her childhood abuse required both psychoanalytic and embodied therapy that addressed developmental needs and relational processes. Jodie needed to feel the mutual interaction of touch within her early self-states and childhood traumas.

Her 24-year-old self-state required a different form of treatment. Jodie's violent assault and rape was a single-event trauma that created decades of chronic consequences for her. For Jodie, at this early stage of therapy, her college trauma needed to be processed more in nontouch psychoanalysis for us to work through many of the memories, emotions, and embodied flashbacks she was having in and outside of sessions. Psychoanalytic talk therapy would have reduced the intensity of her flashbacks over time, and the forms of embodied therapy we were engaged in would have then been more effective in addressing her college trauma. In Chapter 10 I will detail the embodied transitional and progressive work that helped to transform her college trauma. In this regressive phase of the work, the inclusion of touch, if it occurred at all, needed to be primarily contact comfort.

An important part of the therapy was to first learn how to separate the childhood and college traumas and then to work on them somewhat independently. This eventually led to Jodie's choosing when to focus on one or both. However, her ability to make that choice was limited in this phase of the work because of the intensity of the college trauma. She was often not able to tolerate touch when the intense feelings and memories of being assaulted and raped surfaced. The problem was that she could not always recognize or tell me when she had shifted from her childhood self-states, which wanted touch, to her adult trauma, which wanted minimal contact. Often she would start a session focused on her childhood traumas and the effective forms of touch we had established. However, a specific touch during the work could shift Jodie into her college trauma. This led to some misattunements on my part that left both of us dealing with our own disruptions. To help work through this phase, we added regular phone sessions the day before a body session so we could talk about what was going on for her and what self-states might need to be addressed in the next day's session.

In a presentation of this case in 2017, I said that if Jodie had only experienced her adult trauma in college I might never have touched her. If her treatment had included embodied therapy, the work would have been confined to holding hands, sitting shoulder to shoulder on the couch, and possibly, eventually, some work around her own embodied agency. My rationale for taking this position was that work within trauma that carries that level of emotional and embodied intensity is best approached within a more symptom-focused treatment designed to help the patient reduce the intensity, duration, and frequency of their trauma flashbacks.

However, I have learned from patients like Jodie, and Mike in the previous chapter, that there are many patients who want to move beyond that type of work into a full body analysis designed to reclaim their stolen body. Although at times I questioned—and, on a few occasions even regretted—having begun embodied work within Jodie's college trauma, she did not. She told me that there were only a few times in passing that she had wondered if that form of treatment was worth it. Jodie took everything that happened in the work—the good as well as the mistakes and misattunements that activated her embodied flashbacks—as necessary to reclaim her stolen body. She never liked my use of the word "mistake" because she felt it implied that I had done something wrong. She saw my difficulty in sometimes knowing how to proceed as just another part of the work, despite the disruptions it could create for her. Her steadfast commitment to her work was instrumental in giving me confidence in continuing to make informed adjustments to her embodied therapy.

Getting It Right: Effective Work with Jodie's Adult Trauma

The session I will present here started with the usual chair-to-chair beginning. Jody seemed restless, and because I was now more attuned, I inquired as to what was going on. First there was silence, then the beginning of a sentence, a pause, and her answer, "I don't know." There had been no indication this might happen in the phone session the day before, so I was even more confused.

More time on the chairs, more restlessness, and confusion for me: Do I increase contact, move away, stay where I was? I thought the best approach would be more contact or staying within our usual pattern, not less contact or pulling away. With patients who can verbalize, this may not be an issue, but for others like Jodie who do not talk or who say they do not know, it is trickier and requires a deep mutual trust.

I thought about possible touch options and chose hand on shoulder blade over hand on arm. I chose her shoulder blade because I was not sure what was going on for Jodie and I thought that form of touch, which was usually received well by her, could provide comfort and containment. In that session, my choice of touch probably would not have mattered. Any physical contact would most likely have created the same result. At the time, I was unaware of how deeply Jodie had descended into her college trauma memories activated by a nightmare the night before. I thought she was experiencing her child-hood trauma because that had been the focus of the previous embodied ses-sion and what we had processed in her phone session. However, she was experiencing her college trauma, in high definition, with embodied flashbacks and fragmented cognitive memories. When my hand rested on her shoulder blade, Jodie pushed me away, curled up on the chair, and went into her own private space. I felt completely closed off. I sat there for many minutes thinking and observing. I had come to know the different body presentations between the childhood and college traumas, so I was able to discern she was immersed in her college trauma. With that information, I moved from my chair onto the couch so we could be face to face, although Jodie did not look at me. I asked if she was remembering her college trauma. She managed to slightly nod yes.

From what I had learned, when Jodie was in that self-state, she needed me with her. But I was still not sure what type of contact would be helpful. I sat in front of her, silent, just watching and being with her. Then, Jodie opened her hand in a motion that seemed to request mine. I asked if that was what her gesture meant. She again nodded an almost undetectable "yes." I moved closer, sitting on a footstool, and she embraced my hand. At that point I realized what might be going on and spoke with my analytic voice: "I've been wanting to help you avoid feeling what you are now feeling. I've wanted to provide comfort. Now I realize you have to use my comfort while you feel this. You have to be able to remember and feel your assault while I am here with you in support. I will be here with you, holding your hand." She nodded another almost undetectable nod and then immersed herself into the awfulness and terror of her assault while I watched and held her hand.

Jodie moved into a fuller immersion of her 24-year-old college trauma. Her internal remembering of that horrible night was communicated to me and witnessed through her embodied flashbacks. Her body was at times convulsing and other times trembling. Each body shift seemed to connect to a different memory of her assault. She ended her insufferable remembering silently curled up in the chair with tears running down her cheeks while still holding my hand. For my part, I had been both a witness and physical presence in those memories of her trauma. Watching her was almost intolerable, although certainly not as bad as what Jodie was experiencing. The session ended with comfort contact and completion touch: hand holding, a mild embrace, and enough processing to help ground her in the here and now so that she could drive home.

That session was one of many pivotal moments of physical contact in our work. During later processing, Jodie said she believed it would not have been possible to have fully immersed herself in ways that helped connect specific events from that night to certain body sensations without her awareness of my presence through holding my hand. Throughout the work on her college trauma, I never heard a full verbal narrative of the assault and rape. Jodie could not provide one given she had been drugged and some parts of the assault were unavailable to cognitive memory. However, in that session, her body did provide both of us with many of the missing parts of her experience.

That session also forged new connections between Jodie and me within her 24-year-old self-state. It helped me understand how to become more attuned with Jodie's college trauma. This session also marked a turning point in Jodie's work on her college trauma as she was now becoming able to internalize me in her trauma memories. She was beginning to take our connection within her trauma and make use of it as a containing function when her trauma memories were activated outside of the sessions. That session also led to even more intense work and transformations for Jodie about her college trauma.

I Want to Be Held, Not Touched

Following the session just described, the work on Jodie's rape and assault continued to be revisited and reworked within a regressive phase. Her college trauma would often be activated or intensified by something outside of our sessions, such as a report of a local assault or rape in the news. Occasionally, she would find herself near the location where her assault had occurred, which would intensify her embodied flashbacks. However, she now had someone in me, her analyst, whom she could disclose those moments to and then verbally address the embodied sensations and flashbacks using our therapeutic physical connection. Jodie was also using her phone sessions to tell me what she was experiencing the days before an embodied therapy session. This helped me plan our embodied sessions ahead of time and allowed Jodie to actively participate in the planning. She was also developing an increased ability and confidence in directing the physical contact in sessions.

The session I will describe next occurred the day after I received a call from Jodie. She was in a state of terror after hearing on the news about an abduction and rape in a shopping mall she often frequented near her home. The news had activated the memories of her assault and rape in ways that were now more available and intense. We scheduled a session for the next day, which was a Friday. Given the intensity of the flashbacks, I did not want her dealing with them alone all weekend. I thought that would feel too much like the weekend she spent alone in her dorm room following her assault and rape.

I learned from Christopher Bollas both through lectures and writing (Bollas, 2013) about the importance of increasing the frequency and extending the length of sessions as needed when a patient is moving into the throes of a breakdown. I felt that Jodie was quickly moving into a deep trauma state and maybe even a breakdown, which required a form of session that Bollas had developed.

In our phone conversation, I was struck by a comment Jodie made: "My 24-year-old self wants to be held but not touched." I was able to see how this "held but not touched" form of contact had been important to her in the session I described earlier where she opened her hand and wanted me just to hold it. That had provided containment and empathic connection, whereas more touch would have felt intrusive within her college trauma flashback.

The next session we had was 3 hours long. Jodie and I first planned out the structure, and then I consulted with colleagues to ensure the work had been well thought out. The 3 hours would provide approximately an hour each for a beginning, middle, and end to the session. We both sensed that the college trauma had surfaced in a new way that required a structure that would allow Jodie all the time she needed to remember, feel, and explore that trauma.

First Hour

Jodie and I anticipated that she would initially want to collapse into a more intrapsychic experience, wanting me available but in the background until she could make more use of me later in the session. The physical contact in the first hour would involve forms of "holding not touching." Jodie spent almost the full hour working within a more intrapsychic space and using our physical contact for grounding whenever she wanted reassurance I was still with her. The physical contact during this phase consisted of us sitting next to one another on the couch, holding hands, shoulder to shoulder. Occasionally, I initiated a firm but gentle squeeze of her hand to remind her I was attuned and available to her.

At one point, Jodie's shoulder began to twitch, and I placed my hand on her shoulder blade. This misattunement interrupted the flow of her internal space, which was not productive. Unlike in the past, this misattunement did not shift her out of the work. Rather, she merely moved her shoulder to signal nonverbally that my touch was not helpful. In the past, I would have over-corrected and pulled too far away, probably completely disengaging my touch. This time, I merely removed my hand from her shoulder blade but continued to hold her hand. My wanting to create a deeper connection within her embodied flashback had contributed to my touching her shoulder. I reminded myself that Jodie wanted to be held, not touched, and that my attentive presence was all she wanted or needed from me in that moment.

As the session progressed, Jodie's body movements increased, and she began to put some words to what she was noticing in her body and memories. I joined her in her memories. She slowly provided details of her assault, saying things like, "I can see his face." A few more minutes of silence and then she said, "He was so angry." A few minutes later, "I couldn't breathe." And a final sentence before Jodie again went silent: "He could have killed me." I refrained from saying anything. I sat with her, noticing her body movements and making my own private associations about how they linked to her trauma until she was ready and wanted to engage more with me. Near the end of the first hour, Jodie asked if she could put her head on my shoulder, which I agreed to. I resisted the impulse to move more into contact comfort such as touching her face or stroking her hair. Those were types of touch that were helpful within her childhood traumas but not in this 24-year-old trauma in which she wanted to be held but not touched.

Second Hour

The second hour began to take on a more relational tone as Jodie wanted more connection with me. There was more physical proximity as she asked if I would hold her. I placed my left arm around her, and she placed her right arm around me. Eventually, I gently touched her arm and hand and she occasionally touched mine. We spent the hour holding hands and at times engaging in a hug as we processed some of the 3 years of work that led to that session and the work in the first hour of the session. In our processing, two things stood out for her: Jodie did what she had to do to stay alive, and the attack was more violent than perhaps she had ever realized. She talked about remembering that her entire body was sore for the next several days afterward. She also now suspected that she had been more dissociated than she had realized and that this would be hard to know because she believed she had been drugged. She now thought that she maybe had even been unconscious or passed out. She was now certain he had choked her and that was why she continued to have issues with being touched around her neck. She also made a link to moving into a freeze response that night and compared this to the way she froze when she had been abused by her grandfather.

Third Hour

In the last hour, I was surprised when Jodie's body began to feel more relaxed and she asked if we could move into the types of touch we used in working with her childhood trauma. I was cautious about the shift from holding to touching, but Jodie assured me that felt like what she needed and could use to end the session. Her head was still on my shoulder, and I asked her if I could place my hand on her head. She nodded. I watched her as she rested under the blanket in a state of relaxed exhaustion. Occasionally, we continued to process what we each had been noticing during the first 2 hours of the session. What seemed to be staying with both of us was the level of violence in her assault. The session ended with a completion hug. The 3 hours had felt like 90 minutes. The potential breakdown had been transformed into a breakthrough (Bollas, 2013). Following that session, the work within Jodie's college trauma shifted from the regressive into a transitional phase leading into progressive work that will be detailed in Chapter 10.

References

Bollas, C. (2013). *Catch them before they fall: The psychoanalysis of breakdown*. Routledge. doi:10.4324/9780203069547.

Jodie

Mind and Body Integration

Following the work described in Chapter 9, the focus on Jodie's college trauma shifted into a transitional phase that began to integrate with the work on her childhood traumas, which was already well into a progressive phase. Not all patients who complete embodied therapy in the regressive phase choose to continue work in the transitional and progressive phases. Many are satisfied with having reduced the associations between various forms of touch and their past traumas. Jodie, however, was motivated to move beyond not being terrified and suspicious of various forms of touch and wanted to experience touch that was enlivening. I was also willing to move into that phase of treatment with her. Together we entered into a progressive phase that would transform the way her body responded to initiating and receiving touch without fear of her traumas.

Throughout the transitional and progressive phases, the embodied sessions continued to be structured in a predictable, consistent routine that helped Jodie slowly become more curious and observant of her body from both intrapersonal and relational perspectives. One new addition to the structured routine became working with embodied processes while sitting beside one another on the couch. That provided a less cumbersome space than the two large armrests that separated us on the chairs. The armrest had been an important feature in the regressive phase that helped Jodie feel a solid boundary between our bodies when an embodied trauma flashback was activated. In the progressive phase, such a need for a concrete boundary became unnecessary because Jodie was no longer shifting into intense trauma memories that created anxiety around touch.

To accommodate the extra time needed to work within the progressive phase on both her childhood and adult self-states, we extended our sessions from 50 to 90 minutes. We continued to have two embodied sessions a week with phone sessions to process that progressive work. The structured routine of the embodied sessions consisted of approximately 15 minutes in one chair, followed by 15 minutes in the other. This was followed by 20 minutes on one side of the couch followed by 20 minutes on the other side so that we could work on Jodie's experience from both sides of her body. The final 20 minutes were spent in completion touch, hand holding, and processing.

DOI: 10.4324/9781003215745-11

The sessions now addressed both Jodie's child and adult self-states, sometimes integrating the two within the healing and transformative work of the progressive phase. She continued to have days during which the focus would be primarily on one self-state, but increasingly more sessions contained multiple self-state experiences. There were also still times when her college trauma would inhibit her body's trust of progressive physical contact, even though cognitively Jodie trusted me and the embodied work. However, she was no longer overwhelmed by her trauma memories and could verbally tell me what was happening in her body.

Jodie used the combination of chairs and couch to focus on more progressive forms of physical engagement. She wanted to increase her abilities to initiate and receive touch and specifically to move beyond feeling relieved that touch did not activate a trauma memory to finding pleasure and enjoyment in initiating and receiving touch. Jodie was not trying to provide me with comfort or enjoyment in her initiations of touch but, rather, she wanted to push through her anxieties about touching another person's body, specifically a man's, while remaining fully present.

Progressive Childhood Trauma Work

In the first chair, Jodie was more focused on how her childhood issues created difficulty in feeling that her touch was not "dirty." After initial silence and time spent in her own intrapsychic space, she would spend time practicing progressive touch. The beginnings of this progressive work had begun in year 2 in the regressive phase when Jodie experimented with the interplay between our hands, touching my arms, and later placing her head on my shoulder. These forms of touch were now being revisited without her fearing they would activate her traumas, so she could now be more present and curious about them.

Jodie was now able to contrast years of anxiety around touch with the calmness she was feeling. She spent time touching my hands, arms, and face and experimenting with various forms of touch and pressure. Her touch of my shoulder would move into a completion touch hug before the shift to the other chair. She contrasted the hug she wanted to give me at the end of this part of the session with the hug she was forced to give her grandfather at the end of an abusive visit. I began to expand my use of touch as well, placing my hand on her cheek and touching her hair. These forms of contact comfort created for Jodie a new form of relational engagement that moved her even deeper into discovering what empathic touch would have felt like in childhood. For several weeks, she rested within these moments in ways she said felt like she was receiving the comfort and connection that should have followed her abuse instead of having been left alone to deal with the aftermath on her own.

In this progressive work, Jodie spoke of how the sensations of skin-to-skin contact, without feeling anxious, was a new experience and helped her to both relax and integrate her childhood trauma experiences. She now began wearing tank tops to every session providing more access to her uncovered shoulders, something we processed. Jodie was reclaiming her ability to enjoy simple physical contact with a trusted other in ways that had been stolen from her. She could now believe that there was nothing bad in her initiating and wanting touch not only in our relationship, but in her personal relationships as well.

Progressive College Trauma Work

In the second chair, Jodie's touch incorporated a more adult-to-adult focus that had been absent and unavailable to her since her college assault. The body areas and forms of touch were similar to those in the first chair, but the emphasis was on being present in the here and now within the adult-to-adult therapeutic relationship. Jodie worked on reclaiming a full attentive presence to physical contact within her adult mind and body rather than becoming mentally detached from the touch.

On the couch, that same sequence occurred, with side one focusing on her childhood and side two on our adult-to-adult therapeutic relationship. Jodie began to take in and feel in her body what she already had come to believe cognitively: that her initiation of touch with me did not lead to my sexualizing, objectifying, or abusing her. Slowly and over time, Jodie became fully present and comfortable with her ability to both initiate touch and to receive mine.

Jodie's embodied therapy within the progressive phase incorporated many other aspects of both intrapersonal and relational forms of exploration, too many and too nuanced to detail here. However, there were several specific forms of engagement that stand out as instrumental in Jodie's embodied transformation that I will now describe.

Synchronized Breathing

In year 3, synchronized breathing became another way of creating embodied attunement, first as part of trauma work and later within the progressive phase of treatment. The origins of this breathing work occurred in a Monday session following an extended family vacation Jodie had been on with her parents. Jodie's childhood traumas had been stirred up, and she requested that we make more use of a holding embrace during the first part of the session.

We sat within an embrace during the initial silence of the session's routine, which was longer than normal. I noticed Jodie's breathing was short and shallow. I knew the time with her parents had activated her childhood trauma memories, and I was thinking about how I could create a stronger connection without becoming intrusive. I began to match her breathing. Jodie seemed to pick up on my implicit invitation to connect with our breathing, and she followed my lead into slower and deeper breaths. In addition, her body started to feel more relaxed. This became another way we reconfigured her trauma memories at a somatic level without having to use words that would have disrupted her intrapsychic work. Eventually, the synchronized breathing became an important part of her progressive work.

This breathing seemed similar to some forms of breath work in yoga. Over time, it became a form of attunement that often occurred involuntarily and created another form of wordless connection between us. Jodie's ability to make use of our breathing work outside of her sessions was remarkable to us both. Her performance in many of her physical hobbies, including aerobic activities, improved as she was able to maintain deeper breathing. She believed that in the past, an elevated heartbeat had activated somatic flashbacks of her abuse and that this led to shallow breathing. Her ability to now focus on deeper breaths seemed to break the link of an exercise-induced rapid heartbeat to her past traumas.

Neck Work Revisited

In Jodie's treatment, we had suspended any physical work around her throat area because it activated embodied memories of being choked by her attacker. In the transitional phase of the work, we were able to address her body's instinctive reaction to being touched near her throat and to create new positive sensations in the progressive phase.

The work on her neck also illustrates how sustained bodywork is often necessary to develop the level of trust and body familiarity required before work can occur on certain specific embodied memories of trauma. As described in Chapter 9, my premature attempts to address Jodie's neck issues resulted in intense embodied flashbacks. This part of her assault could only be dealt with following over a year of combined psychoanalysis and embodied therapy that addressed other parts of her college trauma. In Jodie's case, embodied work on her neck would not have been possible within a brief embodied therapy described in Chapter 5. She needed the earlier work to develop the level of trust and body familiarity between us to allow her to confidently move into a transitional phase during which she could make use of work on her neck.

In the work on the couch, I began to notice that in our routine, there were certain positions in which my thumb was closer to her neck than it was when we were in the chairs. I also noticed that Jodie was not moving away, and her shoulders were not turning defensively inward as had occurred in the past. Rather, her shoulders moved outward, almost as if to invite more touch around her neck area. I noted that, but did not change the way I was working for several more weeks. I was committed to not making the same mistake of moving too soon into neck work around her throat.

Over several sessions, I watched Jodie's body become more used to the proximity of my thumb near her throat and the new opened rather than closed response of her shoulders. I then brought what I was noticing into the processing in our phone sessions. Jodie said she was also aware of this subtle but significant shift in her shoulders. In processing, we both felt that the timing was better now to move into more work on her trauma of being choked. In a session in which Jodie was anticipating the shift in my touch, I positioned my thumb to make brief contact with her neck. Her shoulder twitch informed me about her embodied anxiety, but her shoulders did not collapse inward. Rather, they stayed back and open. Her embodied response helped me to decide to allow my thumb to rest on the side of her throat for a few more minutes as we sat in silence before I moved my thumb back to her shoulder. In processing the next day on the phone, Jodie said the touch felt "OK" and that her only issues seemed to have been around its "newness." She also said she wanted us to slowly continue to work on her neck. Over time, we realized that like every other embodied trauma memory we had addressed, once Jodie's body became accustomed to the consistent routine, we could then shift into touch on the throat area of her neck.

For many sessions, the work on Jodie's throat area began midway through the session and was limited to my thumb resting on the side of that part of her throat. Eventually, she became comfortable enough with that sensation that she began touching my neck, and I mirrored her hand movements with my own hand on her neck. Jodie was able to reach a point where she could even gently squeeze my neck in the throat area and feel my safe correlating pressure on hers. One day after a session of prolonged neck work, Jodie said in our processing, "No one has ever been able to touch my neck like this since my abuse." This was another part of her embodied therapy that led to changes in her personal life. Following that work, Jodie found that she and her partner could be more intimate within the neck area. In addition, she found she could now wear clothing that fit snugly around her throat. This work also complemented and expanded on the earlier work around her breathing during physical activity.

Embracing Anger

Similar to having suspended physical work around Jodie being choked, we had moved away from embodied work on her anger and aggression following my early and poorly informed attempts at hard techniques within somatic mastery and modulation. Within the transitional phase that occurred later in therapy, Jodie could now tolerate the anxiety that feeling angry created in her. Her anger had never been welcomed in her relationships with her parents and created ruptures that often took days to repair. During her assault, she believed any aggression toward her attacker could have put her in more harm, perhaps even to the point of being murdered. She may have been correct. As a result, her anger had become split off and only available in the service of others.

The transformative and progressive work around anger was reintroduced into Jodie's treatment in a way I had never worked with anger before. In my years of body therapy, anger was generally worked on using hard bodywork techniques such as the patient hitting a mat with a tennis racket or rolled up towel, or the patient and therapist standing facing each other and pushing against one another. Jodie's work on her anger took on a unique form and is one I have added as a possible option in some situations in which the anxiety about anger includes the patient's fear of a possible rupture of the relationship as occurred in their childhood. For Jodie, given that her anger issues originated in both childhood and in her assault, the work had to account for both of those parts of her.

After Jodie had worked through many of the issues around both her childhood and college abuse, her anger around both traumas seemed to become more available to her. One session, Jodie arrived in a different mood and said she was unsure what was going on for her. We began the standard routine and only began to address this "different mood" on the couch in the more here-and-now adult-to-adult work. Jodie talked about her anger at her grandparents for the abuse and her parents for not doing anything about it. She talked about her college assault and how much was taken away from her by that attack.

As she was speaking, I noticed she was squeezing my hand, and eventually I began to squeeze back. Jodie continued and said she was worried about my reaction if she became angry. Would I move away like her parents had? My reassurance that I would stay with her in her anger helped her to continue talking about and then feeling her anger. After doing that, she shifted position and initiated what could best be described as a bear hug that both expressed and contained her anger. I responded with a containing bear hug. What made this different from anything I have experienced in an embodied session was that the hug was not a form comfort for her. It was one of anger and power, with Jodie and I pushing hard against one another's shoulders. In processing later, Jodie said the hug was her way of asking without words, "Are you still connecting with my anger?" My reciprocity with the firm embrace was my "yes" answer.

I was trying to stay with and match Jodie's adult strength. She occasionally relaxed the embrace and rested in that space. She also talked more about her grandparents, parents, and attacker and then moved back into a powerful embrace. This back and forth process occurred for close to 30 minutes and ended with Jodie's head on my shoulder as we processed.

Jodie said that she had always worried her anger would push people away or get her hurt and that she never could seem to feel it. I told her I found her move to an angry embrace a brilliant way to both feel her anger and power while actually having her and me pushing closer together rather than further apart. Anger in her childhood was never welcomed by her parents and led to punishing distance in which they would ignore her for hours. In addition, her belief that fighting against her college rapist would have resulted in more violence toward her made her afraid that any forms of aggression from her could end in physical harm. I now understood that my use of traditional forms of bodywork around anger were not going to be effective for her because pushing against me activated both her childhood relationships with her parents and her college trauma. Conversely, pushing toward one another in the bear hug permitted her to feel anger and aggression without the traumatic fears of emotional rejection or physical harm.

The Sound of a Heartbeat

On the couch, Jodie discovered that if she rested her head on my chest in a certain way, she could hear my heartbeat. In my work with patients, and in my own bodywork, I had never considered how listening to the therapist's heartbeat could evoke and create a sense of embrace. In Jodie's case, it created a shift into an intrapsychic space that she described as the type a baby probably feels with a loving and protective mother. She added that listening to my heartbeat created a sense of relaxation and a sacred space that she had never felt.

When Jodie was listening to my heartbeat, there was little conversation. My function was usually to observe and engage in ways that seemed to provide connection without being intrusive. I would notice how various parts of her body would gradually relax. For example, her arm around my stomach or her hand holding mine eventually would collapse into what can best be described as the way a child's arm or hand looks in a fully relaxed moment resting on a caregiver. I also noticed shifts in her breathing and would often match them.

Listening to my heartbeat became a part of the routine on the couch. In our processing, Jodie and I tried to find ways of describing these moments. We compared it to Buddhist meditation, a spiritual experience, and even an intrauterine sensation, but none of these seemed to capture the experience. What I believe limited us in describing it was that it occurred within a combination of psychoanalysis and embodied therapy. In this space, Jodie was able to integrate and consolidate her years of work within multiple self-states in both modalities. My heartbeat was being used not only for containment but to allow her to move deeper into a part of her core self. Within the sacred and safe space that we had created, she experienced what it was like for her to enjoy both psychic and embodied peace and resting.

The combination of long-term embodied therapy and psychanalysis provided Jodie with opportunities to relate to me and my body while also developing a new relationship with her own body. Her active participation helped her deepen her capacity for bodily agency. She was now able to initiate touch without fear of me turning the interaction into something abusive or sexual.

She was then able to take this work into many of her outside relationships, in which she began to feel more comfortable with physical contact with trusted people in her personal life. In addition, many of the scenarios that would previously have activated her trauma had been all but extinguished. These included feeling anxious when going outside at night alone; fear of being attacked in parking lots, public restrooms, or stairwells; and passing certain parts of the city that reminded her of her assault.

An additional change that Jodie found remarkable was that her IBS had been alleviated. After years of struggling with medicines and doctor's visits, her stomach was relaxed. Even in sessions her stomach no longer made any noise. Jodie was relieved that she no longer needed to worry about whether there was a restroom nearby whenever she went out.

A Final Addition to Jodie's Therapy: Integration and Unintegration

When Jodie's embodied therapy for both her childhood and college traumas was firmly in the progressive phase, she began describing what we called a full body integration in which all of her self-states were available and being felt simultaneously. I believe her years of embodied therapy combined with psychoanalysis had repaired a mind and body split she had endured for many years. This integration at all levels became a familiar and safe space in sessions and created opportunities for Jodie to move even deeper into herself. We used the term "core" in describing the space she seemed to move into as the session progressed.

We decided to place more emphasis on developing that new psychic and embodied resting space. The work required a nonintrusive form of physical connection that could assist Jodie's movement into a deeper intrapsychic space. Initially, there were sessions during which I was less attuned to the type of space she needed. For example, I sometimes worked to create relational connections through eye contact instead of sensing what Jodie needed was limited eye contact.

I began to pay more attention and make use of information such as body position and body movements, breathing, eyes open or closed, and the other ways Jodie interacted with me through touch rather than words. Eventually, I became more attuned and present without interrupting her shift into intrapsychic spaces that were known only to her. I believe a crucial component of progressive work is that some of the experience for the patient remains internal and private. Previously (Novak, 2021), I referenced ideas by Williams (2019) about the patient's right to keep parts of the session, and self, private. He contrasted this with the traditional psychoanalytic rule that patients disclose all thoughts that pass through their mind:

> This ideal is in reality probably unattainable, but it may, in certain circumstances, be undesirable. Many thoughts pass through my mind that

are elusive, poorly formed, or in potential. They might be frightening, shaming, confusing, or plain incoherent. That I must reveal all of them, come what may, as a rule, seems to me a blunt instrument that could expose or compromise my core self leading to further, not less, isolation. We are all entitled to keep certain things private—even as patients.

(p. 3)

Williams revised this rule to mean that "the patient shares all thoughts that pass through their minds, as best they can" (p. 3). He believed that this type of therapeutic space helps "facilitate development of an authentic personality" (p. 3).

In our processing, Jodie would describe to me as best she could her experience of this more private embodied work, and although I was curious and engaged in processing the work with her, I seldom pushed for more information than she chose to disclose on her own. I trusted she would tell me what she felt I needed to know and understand.

Jodie's work within her core self continued to deepen and eventually led to a new experience for her. This was her ability to shift in session from integration into a space of healthy and contained unintegration. It was a place that Eigen (1992) described while making use of Winnicott:

For Winnicott, it is important for the personality to be able to rest in unintegration, to float or drift between organizations, to dip into form-lessness or chaos or nothingness. At this sabbath point of personality, one takes time off from self. It is important to have time between choices, time simply to be. What a relief not to have to be this or that, not to have to force oneself into a particular shape. ... The psychoanalytic holding environment puts the patient's personality on hold, gives the person time to thaw out ... to let each current or tendency make its contribution.

(p. 272)

Through a combination of psychoanalysis and body analysis, Jodie was able to achieve what Eigen described. Our work together had created sacred space that Jodie used to take time off from herself and her traumatic past. In that space, there was no pressure for her to be this or that self-state for anyone, or to stay on guard for a trauma memory that might surface. She no longer feared that her trauma memories would invade her psychic or embodied resting space. She could now be deeply relaxed and vulnerable within her body not only with me but within her own internal world. Jodie had moved beyond relief of her traumas and into embodied enjoyment, pleasure, and fulfillment. In her words, "A beautiful experience."

Detailing the magnitude of the profound changes in Jodie's relationship to her own body and with others loses something through verbal descriptions. This is the essence of an embodied transformation. Symbolization with words has limits. Jodie often used the ellipsis "dot-dot-dot" to convey how the experience of reclaiming her stolen body was impossible for her to put into words. The transformations she experienced during her psychoanalysis and body analysis over 8 years of treatment were extensive. The changes occurred slowly and gradually as part of an informed and disciplined process that included hours of my own individual and group consultations of this work. Movement through the three phases of embodied therapy offered extensive opportunities for Jodie to reclaim and transform parts of herself that had been stolen, all but destroyed, or that had never been known by her.

References

Eigen, M. (1992). The fire that never goes out. *The Psychoanalytic Review*, 79(2), 271–287.

Novak, E. T. (2021). Working in the terrain of the damaged self core. *Transactional Analysis Journal*, 51(3), 241–253, https://doi.org/10.1080/03621537.2021.1950968.

Williams, P. (2019). Isolation. *Psychoanalytic Dialogues*, 29(1), 1–12, https://doi.org/10.1080/10481885.2018.1560873.

Chapter 11

Embodied Work in Psychoanalytic Psychotherapy without Touch

Within the fields of psychoanalysis and psychotherapy, renewed attention to the patient's body has resulted in interest in how the two bodies (patient and therapist) in the room influence one another and create issues of transference and countertransference. All patients and therapists engage in some forms of nonverbal communication, and there is always a mind and body mutual influence, regardless of whether or not these dynamics are addressed directly in the work.

Some patients are apprehensive enough around touch with their therapist, especially early in addressing their trauma in therapy, that engaging in touch would be unwise. However, even in these forms of treatment, addressing the patient's body without touch can provide the person with rich opportunities to understand the many ways their body holds trauma memories.

I have placed this chapter near the end because I believe that even non-touch body therapy becomes more expansive when clinicians have had exposure to and worked within models of physical contact such as the one presented in this book. Therapists who engage in their own bodywork and study theories and models of touch will find they have an enhanced intuitive capacity to link mind and body when working with trauma patients, even if direct touch is not used.

Inviting Curiosity about the Body without Being Intrusive

Traditionally, psychoanalytic psychotherapy emphasizes helping patients become curious about their own minds and unconscious processes, with limited attention to the body. With the addition of nontouch embodied therapy, more attention can be paid to embodied processes in ways that integrate mind and body in the work. Many authors have written about nontouch embodied therapy and clinical techniques. Caizzi (2012) wrote about how the therapist can establish a positive alliance with the patient through making observations or asking questions about "specific parts of the body and body sensations" (p. 172). Smith (1985) spoke of reading a person's body based on the idea that "a person's physical structure is a statement of that person's psychobiological

DOI: 10.4324/9781003215745-12

history and current psychobiological functioning" (p. 70). He also described many types of focused attention on the body using "soft techniques of psychotherapeutic body intervention" (p. 115) that include posture, breathing, stretching, and eye contact, all of which can be useful in nontouch embodied therapy. Ogden et al. (2006) developed a body-oriented sensorimotor psychotherapy approach to work with trauma and the body. Van der Kolk (2014) has written extensively on therapeutic work with trauma that focuses on the brain, mind, and body.

In my early training in transactional analysis, I was taught to pay close attention not only to what the patient said or was feeling but also to what I noticed about their nonverbal signals and their body. This included noticing how and when the patient shifted from one of the three primary ego states (Parent, Adult, and Child) into another. Generally, the shift was from Adult to a more regressed Child ego state or from Child to Adult. Often these shifts were subtle and noticeable primarily through nonverbal changes such as body posture/position and eye contact or avoidance of it. Paying attention to the congruence or differences between language and body is a standard part of transactional analysis practice that, over time, becomes second nature. Clinical observations of shifts in a patient's ego states or self-states are not unique to transactional analysis, as many forms of psychotherapy and psychoanalysis include that form of attention. However, historically, more attention has been placed on observing and interpreting such shifts than on working directly with them.

Many therapists I consult with initially feel uncomfortable with closer observation of the patient's body and movements. In addition, patients often have limited curiosity about their own body, and inviting them into dialogue and analytic curiosity around their body needs to occur gradually, and only after a therapeutic alliance has been established. Making observations about a patient's body or their nonverbal mannerisms should be done with the same care that an observation or interpretation is offered in psychoanalytic psychotherapy. The therapist's training in psychoanalytic psychotherapy along with their own personal embodied work are important factors in determining the best timing and pacing of such comments.

Learning how to remain observant of a patient's body without being intrusive is an acquired skill, as is knowing when to voice such observations. Generally, observing a patient's body should be more subtle than overt so that the patient does not experience being viewed as an object but rather as a subject, with the emphasis on the mutual influence mind and body have on one another. For example, if the patient is feeling anxious, the therapist can observe how the person is holding that anxiety in their body. When the patient is describing a traumatic event, the therapist can observe how the body might be illustrating details of the event. Often this occurs ahead of the verbal narrative, and the patient's nonverbal and body language provide the therapist with an embodied window into the patient's trauma. Over time, these nonverbal signals become sources of information about possible states the patient is experiencing. The therapist can use their observations and understanding of these nonverbal cues to create attunement with the patient's self-states.

I seldom share my observations about a patient's body or nonverbal communications until the person has become comfortable with including their body in the analysis. I have found similarities between the unfolding of dreamwork with patients and the unfolding of nontouch embodied therapy. Many patients begin psychoanalysis with limited if any awareness of their dreams, often saying they do not usually remember their dreams. The same is true of body processes, which many patients report not thinking about or being aware of explicitly.

In my early years as a therapist, I had only a basic understanding of dreams and how to work with them. Then, when I entered psychoanalytic training and worked in supervision with senior psychoanalysts skilled in dream analysis, my understanding of dreamwork and ways of exploring dreams increased immensely. Processing my own dreams in my training analysis also provided me with a patient's perspective on dreamwork that was comparable to the perspectives acquired in my own embodied work.

From my training and personal dreamwork, the dream analysis I did with patients began to shift from asking one or two simple questions that led to basic answers to engaging patients in ways that opened up space between us to explore and experience their dreams in detail. I learned there were multiple ways to understand a dream and that each probably had relevance for a specific moment, issue, or self-state in the patient's life. I also learned how to speak to patients about the importance of dreams. For example, I explained that we don't "have dreams" but that we "create dreams" (M. Apprey, personal communication, 16 September 2016) and that often this is our mind's unconscious way of getting our attention about a certain issue.

When a therapist knows how to consider a dream with a patient, ask questions, and stay curious about the dream, the patient learns how to be more curious as well and about ways to process dreams. Patients then often start remembering more details of their dreams. Working with the first dream a patient brings into a session often sets the tone for how dreams will be processed going forward. This is likely not the first dream the patient has ever remembered, but it is the first they have brought into a session. That probably signals, among other things, that the person has turned to that aspect of their unconscious experience. Bringing in a dream also signals the development of a cocreated experience with the therapist, who has in some way invited that aspect of the patient into the therapy. This dream and subsequent dreams become an area for the patient and therapist to explore as a way to discover the possible multiple meanings of each dream. This acknowledges that every dream is unique to every patient rather than there being a simplistic formula for dream interpretation.

Many of the principles of dreamwork just described can be found in embodied therapy. For example, the significant mind/body split in many trauma patients often results in limited awareness of their bodies throughout life. Patients often find it difficult to describe embodied experiences from the past or even remember how they and others related to their body. As therapy progresses, and with continued curiosity from the therapist, the body becomes more included in the work. Just as with the first dream a patient brings to therapy, there is often a moment when the patient brings in what might be called the first embodied memory. That is as notable and important in embodied work as the first dream is in dreamwork. It signals a shift in the patient's relationship with their body and with talking about it in session. The therapist's abilities to explore this embodied memory will signal to the patient that their issues around their body are in good hands, setting the tone for continued embodied therapy going forward.

An example of this type of first embodied memory of many patients has been haircuts. Patients have gone into great detail about getting their hair cut, describing how they have seen the same stylist for years and how much they enjoy the sensations of having their hair washed and styled. Some express insight around conflicting feelings of enjoying the experience, on the one hand, but also feeling shame for what they worry could be indulging in an inappropriate secret pleasure. In therapy, they begin to understand that their shame is linked to their trauma history, sometimes including an absence of comforting touch in childhood. They begin to feel relief and can engage in guilt-free enjoyment of having their hair done.

Within this form of nontouch embodied therapy, the therapist can imagine not only what the physical connection was like for the patient but also privately analyze the body sensations they have had in similar situations. This establishes a cocreated form of processing focused on the patient's embodied sensations rather than the therapist's. The processing includes exploring multiple meanings and links to the embodied memory being addressed. Similar to dreams, the meaning and links of embodied memories will be unique to each person.

Degrees of Nontouch Embodied Therapy

Working with somatic processes in talk therapy occurs at different levels of complexity and intensity depending on the therapist's abilities and the patient's receptiveness. As noted in the previous section, many patients find paying direct attention to embodied processes new and uncomfortable. Nontouch therapy is a way to introduce working with embodied processes while developing a therapeutic atmosphere that assists the patient in becoming comfortable and curious about addressing their body in treatment. If the patient is receptive to this form of work, therapy may later move into more complex and detailed observations around the body. The therapist should always be gauging the patient's readiness to move deeper or to hear an inter-pretation or reflection about their body or mannerisms as therapy progresses.

As part of early discussions, the therapist may also need to provide some form of psychoeducation relative to including more direct observations about the body and nonverbal expressions. This may include explaining that there are both mind and body issues that may come up during their therapy and that often the body provides information about an issue first that is later put into words. The therapist can explain that along with listening and thinking about what the patient says, they will also be noticing some things about their nonverbal communications and body movements, and that the patient will also most likely notice things about the therapist's nonverbal expressions and body movements as well. The therapist can invite them to ask questions about anything they may notice if they choose and that the therapist might also inquire about something they notice. During this rather brief psychoeduca-tion, the therapist can gauge the patient's level of interest in addressing their body in treatment. The patient's responses can range from sharing how they have already been thinking about their own mind/body connections to a total dismissal and even anxiety about the prospect of paying attention to their body. This initial discussion is also important in developing the trusting alli-ance necessary to work in the terrain of mind and body.

Based on the patient's interest and the therapeutic need, nontouch embo-died work can range from attending to specific body sensations or nonverbal expressions to a more sustained and integrated focus on mind and body. Over time and as the therapy deepens, an atmosphere similar to working directly with touch develops where neither mind nor body are privileged. In certain cases, this integration becomes so substantial that there is a sense of a mind/body amalgamation. In such an experience, the therapist begins to sense even subtle instances in the patient when mind and body are in harmony and when they are more spilt from one another. Over time the therapist develops an intuitive sense of the patient's relationship to their own body and can notice a predictable pattern of movement that correlates to certain thoughts and issues. For example, a therapist may notice how a patient's verbalization of a trauma leads to shallow and anxious breathing, while in other instances body movements such as a reoccurring shoulder twitch can be linked to a specific trauma or self-state and often occurs outside of the patient's awareness. The more a therapist engages in analysis of their own body, the more natural the integration of mind and body becomes in their work with patients. This includes an increase in their intuitive ability to analyze both the patient's thoughts and body simultaneously.

The Embodied Presence of the Patient and Therapist

A similar process occurs within the embodied relationship between patient and therapist. As the relationship evolves, the impact of the therapist's embodied presence on the patient becomes more known in ways that can be analyzed and used in treatment. There are many ways the therapist's embodied presence has an impact on the patient and creates embodied relational connections. These include mutual gaze and even embrace through eye contact, mirroring of body position, and synchronized breathing. These are periods of interrelatedness that contribute to a psychic and embodied resting space for the patient without actual physical contact. For many patients, this form of embodied work will be enough for body transformation. For others, such work, while certainly important and meaningful, will require actual touch because of the level of their embodied trauma.

Of course, the embodied presence of the therapist can also create disruptions for the patient, even in nontouch therapy. The therapist's body and nonverbal expressions can evoke both positive and negative transferences and projections, and all are important aspects of treatment. An example of a negative reaction to my own nonverbal communications may be helpful in illustrating the impact of the therapist's embodied presence.

In sessions, I often spontaneously move my hands as I speak, something one patient used to pay close attention to. In childhood, he had been routinely slapped by his father and told he was stupid. Apparently, at one point I was a bit more animated than usual, and my hands were an active part of my responses. The patient was able to tell me in a matter-of-fact way that my hands sometimes frightened him. From his fearful stare and stiff body posture, I knew that his matter-of-fact comment was not congruent with his internal reaction. I assumed my animated hand gestures were activating his memories of being slapped and beaten by his father. I apologized and committed to being more self-aware of my hand gestures. Following that session, I began noticing when he stared vigilantly at my hands, which signaled that his feelings of childhood abuse were more intense. I began to realize that my hand gestures were not generally activating his childhood traumas, and when his trauma memories were less intense, those gestures seemed to go unnoticed. He seemed only intensely focused on my hands when he arrived for a session already feeling his childhood traumas in high definition. On those days, I became better at catching myself using hand gestures, and the therapeutic correction was that I placed my hands back on my chair's armrests. I also made other adjustments, such as keeping my body in a relaxed posture and sinking into my chair rather than sitting in a more forward position that could feel confrontive. I was also more careful of my interpretations and phrasing so as to minimize them being heard or taken by him as a form of me calling him stupid.

Mistakes in Nontouch Embodied Therapy

An issue for the therapist can be when and how to bring in their observations of the patient's body and nonverbal expressions. As mentioned earlier, most patients are not thinking about their body or the ways the therapist might be observing it. On the other hand, inattention to the patient's readiness or interest in addressing embodied processes can lead to mistakes related to ill-timed observations or interpretations by the therapist. In such instances, the patient can feel caught off guard, which can lead to many reactions from the person, including shame and/or anger or even an intense rupture in the relationship.

McLaughlin (1992/2010) wrote about his own enactment around body issues with a patient he called Mr. E. The patient picked at the periungual skin on both of his thumbs so much that there was actual bloodshed in sessions. This led McLaughlin to comment on the behavior "because I assumed that the physical pain he must be experiencing was surely in his awareness" (p. 171). To Mclaughlin's surprise, the patient had been unaware of his behavior and became visibly upset. In a subsequent session, Mr. E said he "felt caught, shamed, rendered helpless, afraid he was about to be given an actual beating" (p. 171). The patient had been engaging in skin picking since childhood and had been severely punished for it by his mother. McLaughlin's calling attention to Mr. E's behavior created a painful exposure and disruption that took many sessions to resolve.

In my psychoanalytic work with a patient whom I referred to elsewhere as "Jennifer" (Novak, 2008), I created a painful exposure and disruption for her that actually resulted in her leaving therapy for an extended period. Over several sessions, I had noticed that she held and massaged her throat whenever she was thinking or speaking about her childhood sexual abuse, which had involved oral sex. I saw her physical gesture as connected to her abuse and waited over a month before making that interpretation. I assumed correctly that she was not aware that she was engaged in that form of self-soothing in session. My mistake was pointing out the gesture rather than remaining observant and silent. Despite my attempt at timing my observation to the right moment, my words caught her off guard. She found my observation both remarkable and incredibly shaming because she had been consciously unaware she was doing it. While I was hoping the acknowledgment of her gesture would move the work deeper into her abuse issues, Jennifer did not show up for her next session and temporarily ended treatment. On her return, we processed how my attention to her traumatized body had overwhelmed her. She was not interested in linking her childhood abuse to her current issues in any detail, only in generalizations. This became how we worked for several years. A general rather than detailed focus on her embodied trauma was more effective for Jennifer and resulted in her finding ways to reclaim her stolen body at the levels she wanted and needed.

What makes cases like Mclaughlin's (1992/2010) and mine (Novak, 2008) important is that in both instances the therapist spoke about the patient's body before the patient was ready. Both patients were blindsided by their therapist's comments, and in my patient's case, the addition of an interpretation about what her behavior meant only intensified her shame.

Even in the case of Jodie presented earlier in this book, where the treatment was a full amalgamation of psychanalysis and body analysis, I needed to measure when and how to bring things I noticed about her body into a session. An example would be the incident in Chapter 9 when Jodie began wearing long-sleeved winter tops in the middle of the summer during an intense period of work on her college assault and rape. To have pointed this out to her during the session would have been disruptive to her, and I suspect she would have been quite confused about why I was focusing on her clothing. Given the deep state of her embodied trauma flashbacks, she needed to feel I was with her in her suffering and terror rather than analyzing her choice of attire. I held on to the observation about possible links between her traumas and clothing until she appeared ready to process that observation.

Eye Contact

Perhaps one of the more intimate and intimidating forms of nontouch in psychoanalytic psychotherapy is eye contact between patient and therapist. In regressive work, the therapist's eye contact can be experienced as a welcoming and holding parental gaze. As the work moves from regressive to progressive, eye contact will, at times, create a more intimate, adult-to-adult connection. This contact may even contain an erotic quality, signaling therapeutic aliveness that can be important and transformational when processed.

An example from my own bodywork illustrates exploring eye contact both with and without the inclusion of touch and how I made use of my insights from that work in therapy with my patients. With one massage therapist, whom I will refer to as "Jackie," I was able to explore different types of eye contact. This occurred spontaneously one day when we were processing after a massage. Knowing my history, she cut me off midsentence and bluntly said, "You know, you can look at me." I was mildly embarrassed and stunned to discover I was enacting a part of my relationship with my mother, who would sometimes scream, "Don't look at me!" From those interactions, I was conditioned to avoid direct eye contact with women. Jackie knew that history and wanted to help me move through the issue. I stood there, just looking at her while she looked back at me. I must admit it was uncomfortable for me, but not for her. As I tolerated my discomfort and continued to engage in a mutual gaze, I began to notice that I was looking at her but not seeing her. That is, my eye contact was more of a vacant stare without really taking in her or her eyes. Even with her permission and encouragement, I found it difficult to see and take pleasure in our eye contact.

We began working on eye contact before and after each massage. I would also process those interactions with my analyst and take back important information to Jackie that we would then use to adjust our work. Jackie's warm and welcoming eye contact and her reassuring smile provided wordless encouragement for me to relax and enjoy the moment with her rather than fear she would find my gaze lecherous. I was developing the ability to not only look at her but to see her as well. I discovered I could enjoy taking in her eye contact without becoming the overly sexualized, lecherous man I had always feared I might become because of my childhood sexual abuse.

Later, when Jackie and I incorporated eye contact into my massages, the work became infused with even more intensity. I was discovering how gaze, when combined with touch, seemed to intensify embodied responses within different self-states. Over the course of many massages, this work moved through a regressive–transitional–progressive pattern. In the regressive, I experienced a form of loving maternal gaze that had not been available to me in my childhood. Given my mother's own sexual abuse history, I suspect all gazes between us probably felt dangerous to her, as if the gaze would turn sexual, and I believe this was implicitly communicated to me. In that regressed state during massage, the intensity and innocence of my gaze was met by both Jackie's welcoming gaze and physical touch, which created an experience of safe and boundaried connection to her. I was also more comfortable enjoying the combination of eye contact and her touch when experiencing her as a maternal figure.

As we transitioned into a progressive phase, our eye contact and physical connection became more adult-to-adult. My comfort with that would not have been possible if we had not first worked on that form of eye contact without touch. Adding eye contact to the physical massage intensified the connection that again evoked my fears of being seen as lecherous. More processing with my analyst helped me separate my childhood sexual abuse from the new enlivening experience of eye contact and touch with Jackie. I shared this processing with her, and she used the moment to tell me she did not find me lecherous. She added that she had a profound respect and appreciation for me and the work she and I were doing. This relational moment was transformative for me because it was overt confirmation that Jackie found me to be trustworthy within progressive embodied relating.

That work also expanded my understanding of how regressive gaze is less complicated than progressive gaze when combined with physical contact. Progressive adult-to-adult gaze while engaged in touch with a patient seems to be one of the more challenging aspects of embodied work. Sustained eye contact can create intense transference and countertransference, even in non-touch therapy. Including this type of eye contact while working with touch may be beyond the comfort and skill level of many patients and therapists. When I am working in a progressive phase of embodied therapy with a patient, our eye contact is seldom more than brief moments of connection, primarily because it has a tendency to shift the patient out of a more asymmetrical, internal, self-reflective space.

A therapist can also become aware of when either the patient or they themselves seem to be looking but not seeing the other person. This too tends to be a cocreated experience that in psychoanalytic psychotherapy could also be seen as a transference and countertransference dynamic with different meanings in each specific therapeutic relationship. I have noticed a tendency to look but not see the body of patients who have spent years avoiding their bodies. In sessions, my way of looking but not seeing seems to be a form of collusion with the patient's own body avoidance. As already addressed in this chapter, whether the therapist decides to speak to these types of issues or remains a silent but now seeing observer, will be based on the therapeutic benefits of and the patient's readiness to hear such observations.

References

Caizzi, C. (2012). Embodied trauma: Using the subsymbolic mode to access and change script protocol in traumatized adults. *Transactional Analysis Journal, 42*(3), 165–175. https://doi.org/10.1177/036215371204200302.

McLaughlin, J. T. (2010). Nonverbal behaviors in the analytic situation: The search for meaning in nonverbal cues. *American Imago, 67*(4), 487–514. https://doi.org/10.1353/aim.2010.0029 (Original work published 1992).

Novak, E. T. (2008). Integrating neurobiological findings with transactional analysis in trauma work: Linking "there and then" self states with "here and now" ego states. *Transactional Analysis Journal, 38*, 303–319. https://doi.org/10.1177/036215370803800405.

Ogden, P., Minton, K., & Pain, C. (2006). *Trauma and the body: A sensorimotor approach to psychotherapy.* W.W. Norton.

Smith, E. W. L. (1985). *The body in psychotherapy.* McFarland & Co.

van der Kolk, B. (2014). *The body keeps the score: Brain, mind, and body in the healing of trauma.* Penguin Random House.

Chapter 12

Further Considerations and Ongoing Discussions about Embodied Therapy

See Me, Feel Me, Touch Me, Heal Me

I have been a fan of musician Pete Townshend and the group The Who since my adolescent discovery of rock and roll music. Townshend's lyrics always stir emotions and connections in me. As I began writing this book, I also started reading Townshend's (2012) autobiography. Soon after The Who began playing together, Townshend (1966) wrote a one-song mini-opera entitled "A Quick One, While He's Away." Townshend (2012) said that it is his "own story retold in fairy tale" (p. 157) and that the mini-opera "is full of dark reflections" (p. 101) of an abusive time in his childhood when he was sent to live with his grandmother at age 5. Incredibly, when Townshend composed the song, he was unaware that he was addressing his own childhood trauma, instead thinking that the song was an "inadvertent" (p. 159) disclosure of his abuse because the "music bubbled up urgently from my subconscious mind" (p. 101). He said it was "meant to be light-hearted" (p. 159) and that the upbeat, intense music conceals the real meaning of the song's lyrics. A second concealment is that the song is about a little girl, not a boy. The lyrics can easily be interpreted as referring to a young woman because most listeners would find it hard to believe that Townshend was addressing sexual abuse of a little girl. In his autobiography, Townshend revealed that the little girl in the song symbolizes "my imaginary constant friend … a twin girl who suffered every privation I suffered" (p. 102). Townshend wrote that it was that fantasy of twinship that helped him never to feel alone during his traumatic childhood. This surprising, if not jolting, revelation of the song's true meaning destroyed my ability or desire to listen to it, and the song has since been deleted from all of my playlists.

I was not surprised to read that Townshend's and The Who's famous rock opera Tommy (1969), about a "Deaf, Dumb and Blind Boy" (Townshend, 2012, p. 146) was influenced by Townshend's experience of parental abandonment and physical and sexual abuse, which occurred at roughly the same ages as mine had. What did surprise me was a newspaper article (Dawson, 2019) that described Townshend's decision at age 72 to never engage in a full

DOI: 10.4324/9781003215745-13

performance of *Tommy* again because certain songs that infer sexual and physical abuse activate his own childhood traumas. His last full performance of the rock opera was in 2017 when he performed it with lead singer Roger Daltrey at a benefit concert for the Teenage Cancer Trust. Townshend had to leave the stage during the show and could not continue performing songs from the album. That concert was over 65 years after his abuse, and Townshend was still haunted by his childhood traumas.

"See me, feel me, touch me, heal me" (Townshend, 2012, p. 146) is a repeating chorus throughout the opera that represents the inner voice of Tommy. It seems to resonate with the inner voice of many trauma patients I have worked with in my 30-year career. Townshend found a remarkable way to give his Child ego state a way of being heard in the lyrics of *Tommy*. His almost anthemic leitmotif, "See me, feel me, touch me, heal me," takes on an even more profound meaning when heard as the inner voice of Townshend's Child ego state and his longing to be seen, felt, touched, and healed. Obviously, "transform me" would not have had the lyrical smoothness of "heal me," but Townshend's words and rock opera describe many of the challenges that face abuse survivors with embodied trauma.

Like Townshend, many trauma survivors are unaware at a conscious level of how their trauma continues to impact them, if they even remember the abuse or connect it to their body issues. As mentioned in Chapter 1 of this book, the traumatized individual consciously or unconsciously holds on to the possibility of one day meeting someone who can see, feel, and touch their trauma in ways that lead to healing and transformation. Often this person is a therapist, but even in an optimal therapeutic relationship it may take years for a patient to grasp the magnitude of how deeply their trauma has affected them emotionally and relationally. Only after this recognition do they begin to understand how their body has been affected. The patient first needs to develop a deeper understanding of their trauma in talk therapy before engaging in embodied therapy so that the latter can be informed by both the talk therapy and continued processing of the bodywork.

Blind Spots and Therapeutic Collusions around Touch

Multiple theories of trauma all point toward attention to embodied process, but psychotherapy and psychoanalysis seem almost in a state of professional denial about acknowledging that embodied trauma requires direct attention to the physical body, including physical contact. This is regrettable because the trust and safety of the therapeutic relationship provides one of the best opportunities for a patient's body to be empathically related to within a healing and transformative embodied process.

In being seen, listened to, heard, understood, and then touched, the patient can reclaim and transform what has been lost or stolen from them. Psychoanalysis and psychotherapy are in an extraordinary position to be able to offer patients the opportunity to work through issues around physical contact, thereby reclaiming and then integrating body and mind. However, the reflexive aversion to touch and the lack of training in embodied therapy both contribute to a split between what we actually know about embodied trauma and how we treat patients with trauma. Specifically, embodied trauma requires some form of embodied therapy that is not generally available in psychoanalytic psychotherapy.

In psychoanalytic psychotherapy, we know about the Harlow (1959) monkey studies, which showed the importance of maternal contact. The research revealed that baby monkeys preferred embracing a wire frame "mother" covered in cloth over spending any more time than necessary feeding from a bottle attached to a bare wire frame "mother." We also know about how psychosocial deficits create failure to thrive for infants in orphanages worldwide who are neglected and deprived of nurturing caregiver contact. We study attachment theory (Bowlby, 1969) that details issues created for children when forms of both touch and nontouch closeness are not consistently available. These and studies from other disciplines highlight the lasting embodied internal suffering these children struggle with throughout their lives. Although their private emotional suffering often finds an empathic connection in a therapist's presence, when it comes to the patient's embodied suffering, in a metaphorical sense, the therapist has been nothing more than a wire frame.

I absolutely believe that considerable healing and transformation take place in nontouch therapies. Although the embodied work may be incomplete in nontouch treatments, incomplete does not equate to ineffective. Therapists can assist patients in finding ways to attend to the more embodied aspects of their trauma outside of the therapy. But at the same time, I think there are experiences that cannot be fully accessed without some form of physical engagement in treatment. Every therapist has to decide for themselves whether the benefits of embodied therapy with a patient outweigh any risks of working in that terrain.

H. Bacal (personal communication, 29 August 2021) recounted that Heinz Kohut and Michael Balint both offered a paradigm for apprehending and treating traumatic disruption at very early ages. Kohut's idea was that the healthy development of the infant's self begins in the context of a *self-selfobject matrix* and requires the therapist who works with patients for whom this was significantly disrupted to allow for a merger experience. For those who subscribe to this form of treatment, we could say that the inclusion of an embodied self-selfobject matrix offers the patient an experience of sharing their embodied trauma states with their therapist. Bacal noted that Balint (1969) detailed in Chapter 24 of *The Basic Fault* how the analyst could offer themselves therapeutically to such patients in certain nonverbal ways. Both Kohut and Balint, along with D. W. Winnicott, well understood the importance of avoiding retraumatizing impingements in such work.

What these and other analysts could not seem to conceptualize was how to provide and integrate into psychoanalytic treatment the therapeutic experience of embodied connections that certain patients need to heal and transform traumatic disruptions of the self. If embodied therapy is going to become a standard part of psychoanalytic psychotherapy for some therapists and patients, the profession needs to destigmatize many issues around touch in treatment.

Destigmatizing Holding and Touching in Psychological Treatment

I am not naïve to, nor do I ignore that there are multiple forms of boundary violations committed within all helping professions. The arguments against touch in psychoanalysis and psychotherapy seem to be woven into the fabric of those professions, and sealed in by reports and cases of therapists who have sexually exploited patients. Yet cases of boundary violations rarely, if ever, seem connected to embodied therapy that has gone rogue. Rather, most of these cases occur in supposedly nontouch therapies.

A major issue in the continued stigmatization of touch in psychoanalysis and psychotherapy has been the limited advancement of theoretical models and clinical case material presented at professional conferences and in peer reviewed journals addressing the therapeutic benefits of touch. The majority of published material on touch is embedded with criticism and cautions that focus on dangers rather than the possibility of deep embodied transformation. In addition, even the cases that do present a positive example of touch tend to focus on a moment of touch such as a hug or the holding of a hand during a difficult session. In these presentations, touch is implicitly and unintentionally reduced to an à la carte add-on in the moment rather than a theory-based model that can also include more sustained forms of touch such as those outlined in some of the cases presented in this book.

The stigmatization of touch in psychoanalysis and psychotherapy can affect trauma patients in ways that seem to go unnoticed and then unaddressed. Perhaps the most damaging is an implicit, if not explicit, position that the patient cannot be trusted. Often the arguments against touch imply that trauma patients will be confused by, if not incapable of distinguishing between, their abuse and therapeutic physical interactions in treatment. This is often reinforced by the ways a patient's actual fears and distrust of touch are interpreted and framed. In a rather ironic situation, a patient's issues of distrust of their own and other's touch is seen as reason to avoid touch with them. This has a tendency to reinforce their belief that there is something wrong with their touch, that there are good reasons to be distrustful of touch, and that touch is too unpredictable to be engaged in even during professional treatment. It would seem that optimal therapeutic treatment would consist of a therapist who was comfortable with therapeutic touch and who actually believed the patient's exclusive objective was to work through their distrust of touch rather than having an ulterior motive such as seducing the therapist and destroying their career. The therapist's job could then be to help the patient move through their fears and distrust of touch, just as therapists do with almost any other issue a patient brings to therapy, rather than joining in with and reinforcing their fears and distrust of touch.

For the therapist, the stigmatization of touch also implies that they cannot be trusted to hold the therapeutic boundary any more than the patient can. I have always found it odd to think that a therapist in the throes of exploring a trauma experience of physical or sexual abuse with a patient would in those moments be sexualizing the patient. In embodied therapy, the therapist is not at risk of moving into some form of a Dr. Jekyll and Mr. Hyde situation in which the work shifts from embodied therapy designed to benefit the patient into sexual acting out by the therapist who just could not control themselves. Any therapist who engages in their own bodywork would easily learn exactly what their strengths and limitations are in such work and that all forms of physical contact do not lead to sexual arousal or issues of impulse control. I believe therapists already know this from their own daily physical connections in their personal lives. But the professional stigmatization of touch, and reports of boundary violations by therapists wanting to exploit patients or who had not acquired the skills necessary to engage in embodied therapy, create anxiety and discounting of the therapist's own motivations and abilities.

Although I am in favor of and support ethical standards that help prevent the exploitation or revictimization of patients, such standards should not foreclose the possibility of therapeutic touch that is necessary for many trauma patients and is found in embodied therapy. There needs to be a distinction between when a patient's past victimization makes working in embodied therapy ill-advised and therapeutic embodied therapy that identifies with the patient's sense of being a trauma survivor who is ready and wanting to reclaim their stolen body.

Stigmatization of touch in therapy also implies that, given the current incidences of ethical breaches in nontouch therapy, adding touch to therapy will only create more risks of ethical breaches. I argue that the absence of theoretically based models of embodied therapy and limited clinical case material detailing the use of therapeutic touch contributes to an absence of ways to frame and understand touch that is already occurring in therapy. Both nontouch treatments and treatments that are open to or include physical engagement contain boundaries that create safe and sacred spaces within treatment. As already stated, I believe most boundary issues stem from the therapist engaging in unethical practices rather than from an ethical model of embodied therapy. With a reduction in the stigmatization of touch in psychoanalytic psychotherapy, therapists will feel more comfortable discerning whether or not to train in and work with embodied practices.

Touch that Comforts

The profession also needs to address the devaluation, if not outright contempt, for touch that provides comfort to a patient. Such contact is often pejoratively referred to as a "corrective experience" that gratifies a patient's need and is thus seen as nontherapeutic. In nontouch therapy, the therapist's creation of a therapeutic containing environment and even psychic resting space for the patient is met with professional acceptance. Although the suggestion is that such a space is created primarily to help the patient move into deeper experiences of their psyche, it seems rather obvious that it could also feel comforting. However, this secondary aspect of the created space—comfort—is not generally discussed, even if recognized in case discussions. It is also not viewed with contempt. I believe that when physical engagements that feel comforting to a patient are used effectively in treatment, they too are primarily in the service of creating an embodied therapeutic containing environment and resting space for the patient that invites them to safely explore embodied experiences.

In addition, nontouch containing and holding spaces are less effective for individuals who never had an actual sustained embodied relationship with a primary caregiver. A patient who seldom, if ever, experienced a secure physical holding environment has nothing to draw from within the holding environment created in a nontouch psychoanalytic psychotherapy. Their issues of physical abandonment, abuse, and neglect need forms of embodied connection for a more complete transformation. Used in this way, comforting touch is not merely a feel-good corrective moment but an important part of creating space to further explore trauma and body issues.

Therapist Self-Care

As with all work within the helping professions, attention to self-care when engaged in embodied therapy is crucial for the therapist's well-being. Sessions with physical interactions can be quite enlivening for the patient and deeply draining for the therapist. This is partly because the therapist, in essence, does double duty in focusing intensely and interacting with both the patient's mind and body in session. This combination can leave a therapist depleted, especially during body analysis. Psychoanalysts and psychotherapists are familiar with feelings of depletion following an intense trauma session even without touch. Embodied connections that create opportunities for the therapist to share in both the patient's emotions and somatic sensations can be highly therapeutic but quite exhausting.

In my own practice, I have created both a work schedule and a self-care routine that help me address such issues. I tend to keep open the hour following a session that includes embodied therapy and use it for self-processing of the session and to reenergize. When possible, I schedule embodied sessions at the end of the day. In addition, and as most therapists do, I use many self-care rituals in my free time, including engaging in my favorite hobbies.

Perhaps the most important part of self-care when depleted by embodied work is my weekly personal massage. I have found the full attention to a patient's embodied experience can deplete my own sense of embodied vitality. Having spent my week making use of my body in ways that have been in the service of attending to patients' bodies, I need someone therapeutically attending to mine. Massage provides this reparative experience for me. I have been fortunate to have massage therapists who understand this type of therapeutic self-care and are skilled at providing it.

Gender Issues and Cultural Differences

More attention needs to be given to differences based on gender relative to embodied therapy. My work as a heterosexual male impacts my patients differently than if I were another gender. I have also found no standard ways of working within genders because each patient will have a different experience of embodied therapy with their therapist, given their own history and comfort with touch. For example, in Chapter 7, my work with Mike, a heterosexual male, was not something some heterosexual males might have been comfortable engaging in with me. They might have preferred embodied work outside the analysis with a female massage therapist or not to include forms of embodied therapy at all.

Additionally, theory and clinical aspects of treatment need to address variances in cultural norms relative to touch. In the United States, where I live and work, touch is limited in social settings to dull handshakes or some hugs. In contrast, in many cultures, more animated hugs, and even kisses, are a standard part of greetings. However, greater comfort with more social greetings does not necessarily translate into increased comfort or understanding of touch in a clinical setting, and each culture needs to create forms of embodied therapy that resonate with their own patient populations.

Virtual and Phone Sessions

The current Covid 19 world pandemic created the necessity for phone and virtual sessions, which has contributed to what seems to be a professional and perhaps permanent shift toward such forms. This brings challenges to working in embodied therapy that the profession will need to address. For certain patients, the absence of corporeal presence provides a safe distancing that often opens up possibilities of addressing their body. For others, the absence of an embodied therapist in the room forecloses certain issues or makes them more difficult to work on.

One challenge that is rarely discussed is how and when the therapist introduces their own body into embodied sessions. This issue only occurred to me when my analyst mentioned having broken a bone 2 years earlier. I had not known about it because my analysis was being conducted by phone due to the significant distance between our locations. If we had been working face to face, her cast would have been obvious. I wondered, during our phone sessions, whether she should have told me about her injury. I began to think of the issues phone and virtual sessions can create. For example, what if the therapist is pregnant? When does she disclose this to a patient who will not see the embodied changes of a pregnancy? To somewhat address the two-dimensional nature of virtual sessions, I have moved my computer farther away from my chair, which gives patients a waist-up view of me and allows them to see any gestures I make with my hands. The feedback from my patients has been that they prefer being able to see more of me and my body language.

The #MeToo Movement and Fears of Misuse and Abuse of Touch

Perhaps the most common question I have been asked while writing this book has been, "What about the #MeToo movement?" This movement has created space for people who have been silenced to find their voices about issues that for too long have been kept quiet. The question, however, seems to conflate the importance and intensity of this social movement (of which I too am a member) dedicated to bringing into the open all forms of sexual abuse and harassment with therapeutic touch that is informed, disciplined, and in the service of embodied reclamation, healing, and transformation. Therapeutically, I view the #MeToo movement as revealing how many people across the world are in need of the type of treatment the model of embodied therapy outlined in this book can provide. The fact that many people I speak to reflexively refer to the #MeToo movement as a cautionary warning underlines an inherent fear of touch in treatment. To be clear, the #MeToo movement is about individuals who have had their bodies stolen from them; in contrast, embodied therapy is about reclaiming a stolen body within a therapeutic relationship. In fact, the principles and ethics of embodied therapy are aligned with the #MeToo movement.

For readers who are interested in further safeguards, whenever someone asks me how to choose a professional to work with in embodied therapy, I offer these questions to consider:

- How long have you been in treatment with your therapist?
- What training has your therapist done relative to embodied therapy?
- Does the bodywork being considered seem to make sense and connect with what is being addressed in the treatment, and does it seem to fit with your specific embodied issues?
- Is the therapist going to receive ongoing consultation with peers?

- How comfortable would you be speaking about this work with supportive people in your life? If you would feel uncomfortable talking about it, does that discomfort stem from wanting to keep your work private or from fears that the work might be inappropriate?

Many patients prefer to keep embodied work private just as they often keep their psychoanalytic psychotherapy, or parts of it, private. However, this form of privacy should be distinguished from secrecy based on feelings that there is something inappropriate occurring.

Finally, if a patient is uncomfortable with a particular type of bodywork, generally it is best not to attempt it or to wait until more processing has occurred. Too often even empathic encouragement can be experienced by the patient as another attempt to coerce them into doing something that makes them uncomfortable. Having made this mistake myself, I have found that the time processing that mistake would have been better used processing the patient's apprehension of the work beforehand. In addition, if the patient looks apprehensive or confused during a session, it is best to slow down or even stop the embodied work and process what is going on with the patient.

Exploration of Method and Mindset in Training and Study Groups

To more fully integrate mind and body into psychoanalytic psychotherapy, the therapist could benefit from continued exposure to various forms of embodied therapy. This would include more study and collaboration with the many types of body psychotherapy that work primarily with body and somatic processes including Gestalt therapy. Collaborations could also include forms of massage therapy as another way therapists could learn more about touch and the body while providing massotherapists opportunities to better understand and work with issues of transference and counter-transference. These forms of collaborative training will also expand the methods and techniques of touch that therapists can make use of in psychoanalytic psychotherapy.

Because many therapists already touch certain patients at one point or another in treatment, I believe an emphasis on changing the profession's mindset relative to embodied therapy is essential and that touch needs to become more mainstream in treatment. In training and study groups, case presentations could include attention to embodied processes in both nontouch and touch treatments. Case consultations could explore each group member's mindset and thoughts around embodied work in order to increase the therapist's ways of thinking about the work and anticipating what may be needed in future sessions. Additionally, participants could take turns engaging with the case presenter in the types of touch they are contemplating or have engaged in with specific patients. This would provide therapists with more feedback around the embodied work that has been done or is being considered. These consultations could also include ways to process mistakes and misattunements (as discussed in Chapter 6).

Intense and sacred work around the body can be captivating for therapists who choose to accompany a highly motivated patient on a journey to reclaim their stolen body. The possibility of embodied transformation can be an enlivening proposition. However, I have found many therapists have only a basic understanding of such work. The processing of physical contact is often limited to a few basic questions or observations and in many cases overlooked or taken too lightly. The therapist is often unaware of or unprepared for when the embodied work takes inevitable turns into enactments, mistakes, misattunements, and/or the patient feeling that the touch is making things worse. The initial aliveness and enthusiasm can begin to wear off, and the therapist may begin second guessing their choice to include embodied therapy. This is a key reason why collegial support through something like a study group is so important.

Collegial discussions that help therapists envision ways of making use of physical engagement in treatment can lead to unforeseen ways of more fully including the body in treatment. I have heard of many ways that therapists are making use of touch with certain patients and how it has enhanced the work. But with so few articles and case studies on touch in psychoanalytic psychotherapy, there is hardly any way to frame such work within existing theories. In addition, the majority of cases that include touch remain private, thereby contributing to missed opportunities for learning from each other. Inviting more respectful conversations and consideration of touch in treatment could lead to new theory and techniques in working with embodied trauma in therapy.

Embodied Journeys toward Transformation

It is a humbling honor for a therapist to become the first person a patient trusts to accompany them on the journey to reclaim their stolen body. This process usually takes years and requires mutual trust and commitment in order to understand and withstand the intense emotional and somatic sensations caused by sequestered traumatized self-states becoming available in the safe relationship. For some patients, the possibility of embodied transformation after years of silent suffering is what can make the undertaking of this journey bearable.

Individuals show unimaginable courage in deciding after years of private embodied suffering, if not internal torture, to trust a therapist with this hidden part of their self and their body.

Williams (2007) spoke of his own admiration for patients who decide to commit to an intensive psychoanalytic psychotherapy without touch in search of an authentic self:

> Finally, what do we make of the patient who risks embarking upon an analysis and breaking down, notwithstanding the horrors of a psychotic

regression, in a last-ditch belief that finding an authentic self might still be possible? The courage and dignity involved may, to us, be unsurpassed. But my question is: what makes such a painful undertaking thinkable?

(pp. 353, 355)

We can add to Williams's poignant words the patient who commits to a body analysis along with their psychoanalysis. We are faced with their courage and dignity in wanting to dive into the murky depths of body analysis with their trusted therapist in a last-ditch belief that finding and reclaiming their body might still be possible. And then we might ask ourselves, what motivates a therapist to accompany a patient in such a journey? How does the therapist embrace their own trepidation about engaging in such a therapeutic journey? One that involves forms of embodied work requiring an expansion of traditional and comfortable therapeutic frames. Work that by its very nature will include mistakes and enactments that will sometimes take months to explore, understand, and repair. Nonsexual therapeutic techniques that could nonetheless be misunderstood or criticized by colleagues who are unaccustomed to or suspicious of embodied therapy. All with the understanding that the outcome of such work is not guaranteed. How does a therapist come to decide to engage in such deep suffering with the patient and unflinchingly commit to whatever is therapeutically necessary to work at this level? My answer may be overly simplistic, but for me it captures the essence of embodied therapy with trauma patients: An all-in commitment seems to be the only imaginable response to a patient's deep desire to recover their stolen body and to their traumatized self-state's powerful unverbalized request, "See me, feel me, touch me, heal me."

References

Balint, M. (1969). *The basic fault: Therapeutic aspects of regression*. Northwestern University Press.

Bowlby J. (1969). *Attachment and loss. Volume 1 of Attachment and loss*. Basic Books.

Dawson, H. (2019, 13 September). Pete Townshend reveals he is too traumatised to perform The Who's "Tommy" again because of childhood memories of sexual abuse. *Daily Mail.com*. www.dailymail.co.uk/news/article-7462189/Pete-Townshend-says-traumatised-perform-certain-songs-childhood-sexual-abuse.html.

Harlow, H. (1959). Love in infant monkeys. *Scientific American*, 200(6): 68–74. doi:10.1038/scientificamerican0659-68.

Townshend, P. (1966). A quick one, while he's away [Song]. On *A Quick One* by The Who. Reaction Records.

Townshend, P. (2012). *Who I am: A memoir*. Harper Collins.

The Who. (1969). *Tommy* [Album]. Track Records.

Williams, P. (2007). The worm that flies in the night. *British Journal of Psychotherapy*, 23(3), 343–364. doi:10.1111/j.1752-0118.2007.00032.x.

Index